MICROSCOPY HANDBOOKS 34

Contrast Techniques in Light Microscopy

Royal Microscopical Society MICROSCOPY HANDBOOKS

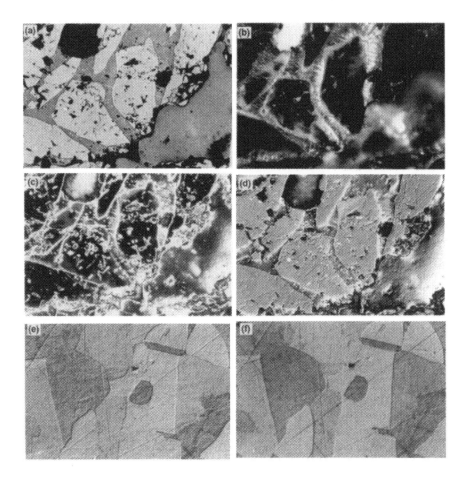

Frontispiece

All the illustrations in this plate are taken with epi-illumination and various contrast modes. The upper four pictures (a-d) are of the surface of a glass-bonded fused alumina grinding wheel; all represent the same field of view and are taken with the x40 objective, the field width in each case representing approximately 250 µm. (a) Bright field. (b) Crossed polars. (c) Differential interference contrast (DIC). (d) DIC but with a different prism setting. The lower left and lower right pictures (e-f) show the surface of a Ni-Cu alloy using DIC with different prism settings to show how the grains appear to be either raised above or sunk below the surface, according to the microscope setting. The field width of (e) and (f) is 250 µm.

Contrast Techniques in Light Microscopy

Savile Bradbury
Pembroke College,
Oxford, UK

Peter Evennett
The University of Leeds,
Leeds, UK

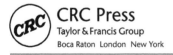

CRC Press
Taylor & Francis Group
Boca Raton London New York

CRC Press is an imprint of the
Taylor & Francis Group, an **informa** business

In association with the Royal Microscopical Society

First published 1996 by BIOS Scientific Publishing Ltd.

Published 2019 by CRC Press
Taylor & Francis Group
6000 Broken Sound Parkway NW, Suite
300 Boca Raton, FL 33487-2742

© 1996 by Taylor & Francis Group, LLC
CRC Press is an imprint of Taylor & Francis Group, an Informa business

No claim to original U.S. Government works

A Library of Congress record exists under LC control number: 00042960
Publisher's Note

**Visit the Taylor & Francis Web site at
http://www.taylorandfrancis.com**

**and the CRC Press Web site at
http://www.crcpress.com**

ISBN 13: 978-1-85996-085-1 (pbk)

Savile Bradbury and Peter Evennett have asserted their right to be identified as the authors of this work in accordance with the Copyright, Designs and Patents Act 1988.

A CIP catalogue record for this book is available from the British Library.

Typeset by Els Boonen, BIOS Scientific Publishers Ltd, Oxford, UK.

Contents

Preface

It is no exaggeration to say that microscopy is in some way involved in every aspect of life in the twentieth century (and no doubt in the twenty-first, too!): in the health sciences, the development and testing of materials, the manufacture of fine electronic devices, the detection of crime, and so the list goes on. Microscopists may thus be called upon to examine specimens of widely-differing types, requiring a range of special techniques. It is in the basic nature of a good modern microscope that it provides an image which contains adequate detail to justify its magnification, using either transmitted or reflected light according to choice. However, for the microscope to fulfil its principal purpose of providing the required *information about the specimen*, a further matter needs to be considered: that of *contrast* between the various features of interest in the image, and between these features and the background. It is not easy to observe and study the transparent inclusions within a living cell mounted in the watery medium necessary to maintain life, the grain structure of a polished sample of metal, or the stresses within a piece of rapidly-cooled glass. These *invisible* characteristics of our specimens must be converted into *visible* features in the image, and this is the function of the *contrast techniques*.

Many techniques for enhancing contrast have been devised over the past century, some of them requiring expensive accessories to the microscope and others easily improvised by the user. We observe from our many years of experience as users and teachers of microscopy that many microscopists fail to make full use of the available techniques, or use them wrongly or inappropriately. In this book we have attempted to bring together information on contrast techniques from a wide variety of sources. Our aim has been to help microscope users understand the basic phenomena on which the techniques are based, and thereby to encourage them to be more adventurous in their microscopy and ultimately gain more useful information about their specimen.

Savile Bradbury and Peter Evennett

Acknowledgements

We would like to express our gratitude to Jeremy Sanderson who kindly read the manuscript in draft and made many valuable suggestions and to Dr C. Hammond for helpful comments, especially regarding polarized light. Needless to say the remaining imperfections are the sole responsibility of the authors themselves.

Safety

Attention to safety aspects is an integral part of all laboratory procedures, and both the Health and Safety at Work Act and the COSHH regulations impose legal requirements on those persons planning or carrying out such procedures.

In this and other Handbooks every effort has been made to ensure that the recipes, formulae and practical procedures are accurate and safe. However, it remains the responsibility of the reader to ensure that the procedures which are followed are carried out in a safe manner and that all necessary COSHH requirements have been looked up and implemented. Any specific safety instructions relating to items of laboratory equipment must also be followed.

1 Introduction

In many mammals, such as the dog, information derived from the sense of smell predominates, whilst in others, such as the mole, both touch and smell are important. Humans, however, gain most of the information about our surroundings from our eyes, so we live in a markedly different perceptual world from most other mammals; for us the eye is our most important sense organ. Complex as it is, the human eye has only limited sensitivity. It responds to that part of the electromagnetic spectrum, between wavelengths of approximately 400–700 nm, which we term 'light'. If all these different wavelengths are present, the signals are interpreted by the brain as white light, whilst if the range is restricted we have the sensation of colour. Short wavelengths represent violet and blue, whilst progressively longer wavelengths give the impression of green, yellow, orange and red. Throughout the whole range of wavelengths the eye is sensitive to changes in brightness, being most sensitive in the green and declining dramatically at the extreme ends of its range. Other properties of light, such as changes in the phase of the waves and changes in the state of their polarization, are not detected by our eyes. It follows that, if we wish to ensure that our eyes respond to any changes imposed by a microscope specimen on the light which illuminates it, then we must make sure that such changes are presented in the final image as changes in brightness and/or colour.

1.1 Why use a microscope?

The eye is not only limited by its response to wavelength and complete lack of response to polarization or phase changes, but also by the extent to which it can resolve fine detail. If a film is used in a camera to record the same scene then a much better resolution of detail may be obtained. It is hard to put a figure on the actual resolution of the eye in terms of point-to-point separation, since this is very variable between individuals of different ages and in differing states of health. If we ignore these considerations the point resolution of the eye is still dependent on several factors. Some are related to the geometry (i.e. the shape) of the object, whilst others involve considerations of the brightness and/or colour of the object. A detailed consideration of the function of the eye in microscopy has been published by Baker (1966) and more recently by Inoué (1986). The quality of the retinal image is also important, since if there is distortion or lack of focusing by the refractive media of the eye (the cornea and lens) then it is obvious that fine detail will be lost. The anatomical structure of the retina must also be borne in mind, since the reception of the image and its conversion into nervous signals is carried out by individual retinal cells of finite size. In the case of fine detail this is accomplished by the cones of the macula (the area of greatest sensitivity in the centre of the retina). Clearly, for two separate points to be perceived as separate, their image on the retina must cover at least two separate cones. Finally, it is important not to ignore physiological and psychological factors which play a part; for example, attention, tiredness and degree of familiarity with the object. Taking all these factors into account, under good conditions at a reference distance of 250 mm, it is usually assumed that objects with a point-to-point separation of 0.1 mm will be seen as separate.

There are many instances when finer detail than this must be studied. In order to do this we need optical assistance in the form of a simple magnifier or, alternatively, a compound microscope. This latter instrument will, under favourable conditions, extend our capability to see details which are separated by about 0.25 µm. The provision of *resolution* (ensuring that the fine detail is present in the image) is the principal reason for using a microscope. Having resolved the detail it is usually essential to ensure that the image has sufficient *magnification* for this detail to be accepted by the eye and brain of an observer, the sensitive area of a TV camera or a photographic emulsion. Such magnification is easy to achieve by combining suitable lenses and will not therefore be considered further here, since it is well covered in other handbooks in this series.

Although it is not relevant to this handbook, it should not be forgotten that the light microscope also provides a valuable tool for gaining qualitative and quantitative information about the physical nature of the specimen. When the instrument is used for this purpose, it is often necessary to sacrifice some of the contrast and resolution of which it is capable when adjusted for maximal resolution of structural detail. For example, in many histochemical procedures, where a chemical reaction is performed on the specimen itself whilst this is on the slide, the presence or absence of a certain colour or reaction product is what is sought. The actual structural detail of the specimen may be very poorly preserved indeed and may be hard to make out.

1.2 The need for contrast enhancement

Once we have resolution, and the image has been enlarged sufficiently for comfortable viewing, then the essential requirement is to achieve sufficient *contrast* between the object and its background for the observer or the recording system to register a difference between the two. This is often summarized by saying that we need *resolution*, *visibility* (i.e. *contrast*), and *magnification*, in that order, magnification being the least important.

Contrast results from the interactions of the specimen with light; some of the effects which the specimen has on light will be detailed in Chapter 2 and include the change of its direction by refraction or scattering, changes in phase, or change in the direction of vibration of the light waves. These, however, are not normally accepted by the eye, by film or by TV cameras. It is, therefore, the function of contrast techniques to convert the results of such phenomena into variations in amplitude and/or colour. A good overview of contrast has been given by Sanderson (1994).

Contrast, then, means the degree to which the object is separated from its background in terms of colour and/or brightness. Because of the characteristics of the eye, in bright light this separation may be as little as 2%, but in poor light the difference (often called the contrast threshold) may need to be increased to 5%, or even more, before the object can be seen clearly. This contrast threshold is also related to the size of the object. If this is very small, for instance approximately 100 µm, then the contrast threshold must be increased even further; in such circumstances there may need to be at least a 20% difference from the background before the object becomes visible. The contrast difference between an object and its background is, therefore, essential for seeing fine detail and it is desirable that this difference be made as large as possible, whether we look at the object with our naked eyes, or with an optical device.

There are several useful analogies which may help the reader to appreciate the concept of contrast. One familiar saying is to liken something which is hard to see as, 'like looking for a black cat in a coal cellar'. Here an object (the cat) has very little difference in colour between it and its location (the cellar), which latter is also often supposed to be poorly lit. The same lack of contrast might apply if one thought about a soldier, wearing white camouflage, standing in an Arctic landscape in the midst of a snowstorm. Yet another example where contrast is lacking is when a transparent object (e.g. a contact lens) is immersed in a clear fluid, such as water in a tumbler. The necessity for the enhancement of contrast is equally a problem when the microscope is used for the study of opaque materials with epi-illumination. The subject of epi-illumination is well covered in the books by Galopin and Henry (1972) and Ineson (1989).

The ability to see resolved structural detail, therefore, requires that we have contrast in our images. Biologists had long ago realized this problem and developed a technique for coping with it. As Hartley (1977) puts it: "Biological microscopists long ago became accustomed to dealing with invisible specimens by staining them, and this practice gained such a hold that the instinctive action of a biologist given a live specimen was to kill and fix it as an essential preliminary, after which the use of dyes could be made to provide the visibility, either in a whole mount or in sections."

There must be sufficient contrast in a specimen so that the observer may see the structural detail resolved by the objective. In many cases the provision of this contrast is far more difficult than the subsequent study and description of the specimen. Some specimens may be naturally coloured, or colour may have been added as a result of some specific staining or histochemical technique. Alternatively, the specimens may be almost colourless and transparent. If the object is coloured, wholly or selectively, then contrast may be manipulated by means of colour filters. Other contrast methods rely on the use of oblique light, either from a single direction or from two or more directions, alterations in the illuminating aperture or, with opaque specimens, treatments of the surface such as polishing, etching, etc.

The above requirements are true, whether the specimen under observation is translucent (i.e. thin enough for the light to pass through it, so-called transmitted-light microscopy), or whether the specimen is opaque to light and is illuminated from the same side as that from which it is viewed (epi-illumination or reflected-light microscopy). The same requirements of resolution, magnification and visibility also apply to the situation in which the specimen itself emits light (fluorescence), as a result of excitation with short wave radiation.

1.3   Assessment of the image

In addition to the ways in which the specimen affects light (detailed in Chapter 2) it is useful to consider briefly those factors which are used by the eye and brain system of the observer to assess and interpret the image. With a microscope, the user is *not* looking at the object itself, but at an *image* of the object. Dictionaries define an image as "an artificial imitation of an object, a replica". In art there is a range of kinds of image, more or less 'faithful' to the object, produced by different techniques (sculpture, oil-painting, photography) and in different styles (realistic, abstract), conveying different messages about the object at the artist's choice. Similarly, in microscopy, we may produce many different images of our objects according to the information we wish the image to contain. We must accept that the image is an artefact, and that it does not necessarily represent 'what the object looks like', unlike normal photographs. The microscopical image is a pictorial representation of some of the information about the object, and is usually the result of a series of manipulations of the specimen, the illumination and the imaging system.

The eye/brain of an observer is very good at the recognition of shapes. We have no difficulty in recognizing and differentiating between triangles with differing angles. Squares are easy to separate from rectangles and circles from ellipses. Even objects with irregular shapes are recognizable and similarities assessed in a qualitative, subjective manner. Similarly, contours are dealt with by our perception, and terms such as 'rough', 'smooth', 'scalloped' and so on are easily applied to their edges. Difficulties do arise, however, when we try to communicate these to others. What exactly is meant by 'irregular' or 'rough' when used in the description of the profile of a microscopic specimen? In recent years the development of TV-based image analysers using powerful microcomputers has made it much easier to approach such problems in an objective manner. Mathematical measurements of areas, perimeters, Feret (or calliper) diameters are now possible, together with many more sophisticated analyses, such as measures of curvature of lines or surfaces and fractal dimensions for assessment of surface roughness. Photometric techniques are available for the measurement of optical densities and it is possible to state with certainty the amount of absorption which is occurring in the specimen, rather than have to make a subjective assessment, as had hitherto been the case. These disciplines, which form what may be termed *quantitative microscopy*, are rapidly developing. We now have the ability to obtain data from which precise objective answers may be obtained to problems which were formerly only subjectively decided by individual observers. With the availability of accurate measures of shape and optical density, the powerful techniques of multi-variate statistical analysis may be applied to microscopical specimens and valid evaluations of changes in experimental situations are thus possible.

Recent developments in the use of computers for image analysis have now extended precise measurements to include colour, by assessing parameters such as hue, saturation and luminance. Here again, as with shapes and contour, the brain of the individual observer (assuming there is no defect in his or her colour vision) is very good at *recognizing* often quite small differences in colour, but without instrumental help we are poor at making precise *measurements* of colour differences.

The final parameter which is often invoked in the description of an object is texture. This gives us many of our visual clues which we use when classifying images, and again, it has proved hard to quantify. It has been defined for image analysis purposes as, "the repetition of a pattern which may vary randomly, in varying degrees, from one position to the next. The repetition frequency may be fine or coarse, the patterns can be simple dots or intricate wavy structures, and they can be anisotropic". Many of the newer generation of computer-based image analysers now incorporate algorithms for the effective assessment of texture in microscopic images.

The complexity and uncertainty of our knowledge of the criteria required for adequate image description is emphasised by the differing parts played in the assessment of an image by the sharpness or definition (related to the outline or contour of objects) and the image detail (often not related to the outline). The presence of detail in an image seems to be of much less importance, however, since if the contrast threshold for the eye is satisfied (as it must be for detail to be perceived at all), then it is noticeable that the observer can often tolerate a very large degree of 'downgrading' of the image in terms of loss of detail. The brain seems to accept this as natural and in many cases it 'fills-in' the missing detail from previous experience. This phenomenon is shown well in some of the illustrations in the books by Frisby (1980) and Gregory (1970). On the other hand, tolerance for loss of sharpness is very low and blurring of an image is rarely acceptable.

References

Baker JR. (1966) Experiments on the function of the eye in light microscopy. *J. R. Microsc. Soc.* **85**, 231–254.

Frisby JP. (1980) *Seeing. Illusion, Brain and Mind.* Oxford University Press, Oxford.

Galopin R, Henry NFM. (1972) *Microscopic Study of Opaque Minerals.* Heffer, Cambridge.

Gregory RL. (1970) *The Intelligent Eye.* Weidenfeld and Nicholson, London.

Hartley WG. (1977) The quest for contrast. *Microscopy* **33**, 231–236.

Ineson PR. (1989) *Introduction to Practical Ore Microscopy.* Longman, Harlow.

Inoué S. (1986) *Video Microscopy.* Plenum Press, New York.

Sanderson J. (1994) Contrast in light microscopy: an overview. *Proc. R. Microsc. Soc.* **29/4**, 263–270.

2 Fundamental Considerations

The image which we see with a microscope is the result not only of the effects of the optical system of the instrument on the light used to form the image, but also of the interactions of the light with the specimen itself. These latter are often forgotten by microscopists, but it is important to consider them, since they form the basis of the rational choice of contrast technique. In many cases, these effects or their consequences on the image may be manipulated by the user in order to enhance or modify image contrast. This may be done either by altering some of the characteristics of the specimen, manipulating the illuminating system at the lamp or condenser and/or manipulating the imaging systems within or after the objective. It is also possible to manipulate the recording or storage medium which receives the final image. Even though a microscope user might not have made a deliberate choice to use a particular contrast technique, one or more of the effects to be described will be occurring and influencing the nature of the image. In order to choose the most appropriate contrast technique, it is essential for the microscopist to understand fully the way in which any particular combination of illumination, specimen, and imaging device act together. It is equally important to appreciate the role of the various conjugate planes of the microscope in image formation, since suitable manipulation of phenomena in these planes will allow alteration of contrast in the final image.

2.1 Light and the specimen

Light and the specimen may interact in any, or several, of the following ways, each of which may affect the image:

- absorption, reflection and transmission
- scattering and diffraction
- refraction and its effects on polarized light
- phase change
- fluorescence

Whatever receiving device is used to record the image, whether it is the human eye or an artificial detector, it must be sensitive to variations in brightness (amplitude) or colour (wavelength) of the light forming the image. These receptive devices are, however, not necessarily able to detect the effects of light which is scattered, or which is refracted, nor are they sensitive to changes in the phase of the light or in its plane of vibration. The results of these important interactions between the specimen and the image-forming light will not register on any of the normal sensors. It is the function of the contrast techniques to convert these concealed effects into amplitude or colour variations, which can be perceived by the sensors in the final image. *Table 2.1* attempts to summarize, for both transmitting and reflecting specimens, the choice of microscopical technique which is best able to generate contrast.

Table 2.1:   Choice of technique

Specimen type	Technique of choice
Transmitting	
Transparent, non-absorbing	
Phase-changing	Phase contrast, Differential interference contrast (DIC)
Scattering	Darkground & Rheinberg, Phase contrast, DIC, Unilateral oblique illumination
Refracting	Phase contrast, DIC, Dispersion staining
Absorbing	
Stained	Bright field
Pleochroic	Plane polarized light
Fluorescent	Fluorescence microscopy
Birefringent	Crossed polars
Reflecting	
Almost perfect mirror	
Slight surface topography	Phase contrast, DIC
Deep surface topography	Bright field, Dark ground, DIC, Unilateral oblique illumination, Stereo microscopy
Surface colour	Bright field
Fluorescent	Fluorescence microscopy
Bireflecting	Crossed/parallel polars
Pleochroic	Plane polarized light

2.2 Absorption, transmission and reflection of light by the specimen

These are perhaps the most fundamental interactions of light with matter, since they must often precede some of the other interactions described later. A good account of most of these will be found in the book by Slayter (1970). When light falls upon an object some of it will be reflected, some of it absorbed, and the remainder will be transmitted, phenomena which are familiar from everyday life. Most of the objects we observe are seen by the light that they *reflect* towards the eye, and their different surface appearances depend on the nature of this reflection. Some objects are transparent, enabling us to observe them by virtue of the light that they *transmit* – wine in a glass, church windows and colour transparencies are obvious examples. In all these cases, the nature of the light reflected or transmitted depends on the *absorption* of light by the object, and may be modified, for example by painting (reflection), or by incorporating a coloured component or dye (transmission).

After a component has been reflected, light will enter an object and may be partially transmitted (passed through the specimen) provided the specimen is not too thick; light which is absorbed may be degraded to heat, initiate some form of photochemical reaction, or be re-radiated as phosphorescence or fluorescence (see Chapter 8). In transmitted-light microscopy, when working with relatively thin specimens, either naturally coloured or those which have been stained, absorption is the principal interaction which provides the contrast. Such objects, commonly called *amplitude objects*, affect the brightness of the light passing through them (see *Figure 2.1*). As far as the production of contrast is concerned, absorption is often the most important interaction which an object may have with the transmitted light. In some cases this amplitude reduction affects all the wavelengths so that the net result is a reduction in the brightness of the object. If, however, only certain wavelengths of the visible spectrum are absorbed (as when an object is stained with a coloured dye), there will be selective absorption of light, resulting in a change in colour of the transmitted light (see *Figure 2.2*). This provides the rationale for staining biological sections and for histochemical reactions which yield coloured end-products. Other objects (e.g. some minerals, exoskeletons of insects) are

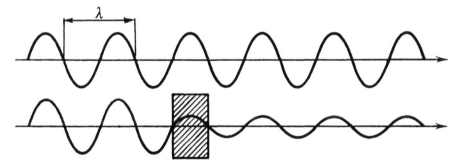

Figure 2.1: The conventional illustration (as sine waves) of two light beams travelling in the plane of the paper from left to right.

λ represents the wavelength, and the height of any point on the curve above or below the datum is the amplitude at that point. The lower beam passes through an amplitude object (shown cross-hatched) which does not affect the wavelength of the light but reduces the amplitude of the transmitted beam.

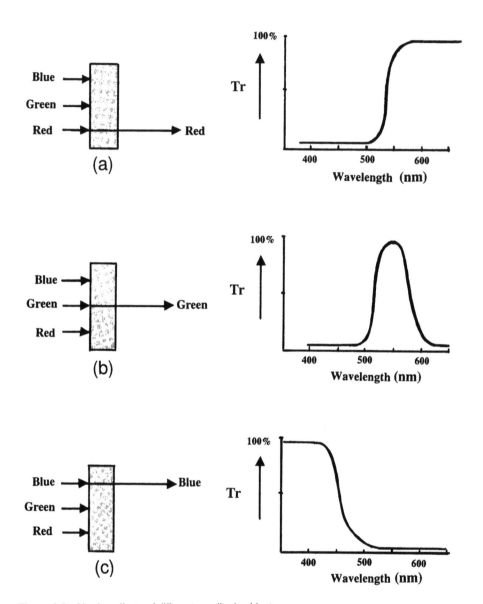

Figure 2.2: Varying effects of different amplitude objects.
   Some amplitude objects affect only certain wavelengths of the light passing through them. Object (a) absorbs the shorter wavelengths, transmitting significantly only wavelengths above c. 550 nm; it appears RED. Object (b) absorbs wavelengths both below c. 500 nm and above c. 600 nm and appears GREEN, whilst object (c) absorbs strongly all wavelengths above c. 450 nm and thus appears BLUE. The axis labelled Tr represents the percentage transmission of the filter.

themselves naturally coloured and again selective absorption provides the major interaction producing contrast.
   When light strikes a surface, some or almost all of the radiation may

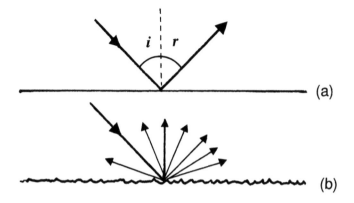

Figure 2.3: Specular and diffuse reflection.
   The upper diagram (a) illustrates specular reflection from a smooth surface. The angle of incidence *(i)* of the light is equal to the angle of reflection *(r)*. In diffuse reflection (b) the light from the incident beam is returned from the surface through a whole range of different angles.

be returned towards the source. If the surface is smooth (i.e. the irregularities are small compared with the wavelength of the radiation), as in a mirror, then we speak of specular reflection (see *Figure 2.3a*). This is characterized by the fact that the angle at which the light strikes the mirror (called the angle of incidence, *i* in the figure) is equal to the angle at which it is reflected (the angle of reflection, *r* in the figure). If the reflecting surface is rough, then the light is returned through a whole range of different angles and we speak of diffuse reflection (see *Figure 2.3b*). Reflection forms the basis of epi-illumination in microscopy.

   The ratio of the intensities of reflected radiation to incident radiation is important, as it has a prominent role in affecting the contrast of the image formed by reflected light. The ratio is often called the reflectivity of the surface. It is related to the angle of incidence, the degree or otherwise of polarization of the light and the properties of the material at the surface onto which the radiation falls. There may also be variation according to the wavelength of the incident light. If the material is opaque, reflectivity is often high; with metals over 90% of the incident light may be reflected. Transparent materials, such as glass, many crystals and water, transmit the bulk of the incident radiation and reflectivity is therefore low. The reflectivity for an air/water interface and an air/glass interface would be approximately 0.02 (2%) and 0.04 (4%), respectively. Although this low reflectivity of air/glass is not of great value in microscopical examination of such surfaces, it is nevertheless important when considering the operation of the microscope lenses themselves, which contain many air/glass interfaces. In complex lens systems, even such a low reflectivity, occurring many times, can seriously degrade the contrast of the image produced. Accordingly, steps are now taken to reduce such unwanted reflection even further. This may be achieved by vacuum evaporating a layer, or layers, of some substance, such as magnesium fluoride, on to the glass surface. The thickness of such layers must be carefully controlled. By such means the reflectivity at coated surfaces may be reduced to a value of less than 0.005. An alternative method for reducing unwanted reflectivity in an epi-illumination microscope system used with objectives of low numerical aperture is that used by firms such as Zeiss (termed by them the 'Antiflex' system). Linearly-polarized light is directed on to the specimen by a beam-splitter and passes through a quarter-wave plate mounted at the front lens of the objective. An analyser orientated at 90° to the polarizer is fitted above the object beam-splitter. Unwanted reflections from the lens surfaces pass upwards towards the eyepieces and are blocked from the image by the analyser. Rays reflected from the specimen, however, will have passed through the quarter-wave plate *twice* so that their polarization plane will be rotated through 90° and will thus pass unimpeded through the analyser to form the image. A modification called reflection contrast microscopy, introduced by Ploem in 1975, allowed the extension of the basic approach used in the Antiflex objectives to oil immersion objectives of high aperture by various modifications, including fitting a central stop in the illuminating system (a good review of this technique is to be found in Ploem, 1995).

2.3 Scattering and diffraction

When a beam of light passes an opaque edge it does not produce an absolutely sharp shadow of the edge, but there appears to be some spreading of the light into the dark area of the shadow, as if there is some apparent bending of the beam. This phenomenon (which we now call diffraction) was noticed by workers as far back as the seventeenth century. It was not until the early nineteenth century that it was systematically studied, first by Thomas Young and later by Fresnel and Fraunhofer. Both diffraction and refraction (outlined in the next section) are terms which imply the bending or deviation of light waves. The term diffraction is, however, confined to those instances in which the bending of the light is specifically attributable to its wave-like properties, whereas refraction is used when the bending is at a surface where there is a change in the medium.

In discussion of the generation of contrast in the microscope, the terms *scattering* and *diffraction* can be considered to be almost synonymous. The term diffraction is often used to describe a special case of scattering, in which an object with regularly-repeating features produces an orderly redistribution of light (diffraction pattern). Complex objects, such as the majority of our microscopical specimens, can be considered to be made up of many simpler, diffracting features which, when taken all together, produce an apparently random scattering of light.

In normal vision, observation of the presence or qualities of some objects is due to these phenomena. Otherwise-invisible marks on a car windscreen become most noticeable when they scatter light into your eyes from the sun or from another car's headlights; likewise, fingerprints on a polished tabletop appear lighter than their background, because they redirect into the eye, light which would otherwise have travelled in another direction.

The mathematical treatment of diffraction is complex, but the phenomenon may be explained by the principle first enunciated by Huygens, which postulates that each point along a wavefront may be considered as the source for the origin of a secondary wavefront. From these the position of the ensuing wavefront may be found by drawing a tangent along the envelopes of the secondary wavefronts and its direction is a normal to this. It is now relatively easy to illustrate the formation of diffraction fringes by the use of the very intense coherent beam of light produced by a laser, but the phenomenon may also be seen using waves on the surface of water in a ripple tank (see *Figure 2.4a-d*). *Figure 2.4a* shows a series of uninterrupted parallel wavefronts; *Figures 2.4b* and *c* show parallel wavefronts passing through a narrow and a wide slit, respectively; *Figure 2.4d* illustrates the interference which results from the interaction of two circular wavefronts. In *Figure 2.4c*, 10 or 11 secondary sources of wavefronts are illustrated, although of course we must remember that an infinite number of such series actually exists, together with some of the new wavefronts arising from them deviating into the shadow areas at the ends of the slit. There is not a graded fall-off of the light intensity into the shadow area but, because of the fact that the secondary wavelets are coherent and have special phase relationships with each other, they will interfere to give a series of dark and light fringes. It is worth noting that the phenomenon of diffraction is essential to the process of image formation in the microscope, as was first appreciated by Ernst Abbe in the 1870s.

Diffraction may be used to influence contrast of transparent microscopic specimens, especially the accentuation of borders, by careful manipulation of the conditions of illumination. An understanding of diffraction also is involved in the explanation of contrast formation in dark-ground and phase-contrast imaging.

2.4 Refraction and polarized light

Light travelling in a vacuum has a constant speed (designated by the symbol c) of approximately 3×10^{11} mm sec^{-1}. When the waves pass into a different medium they will travel at a slightly different speed and are thus often deviated from their former straight line (see *Figure 2.5*). This phenomenon occurs at air/glass interfaces and it is by this process that glass lenses work. Refraction will also occur between the specimen and its mountant, or even between different parts of the same specimen. It is expressed as the *refractive index* (RI), defined as the ratio of the speed of

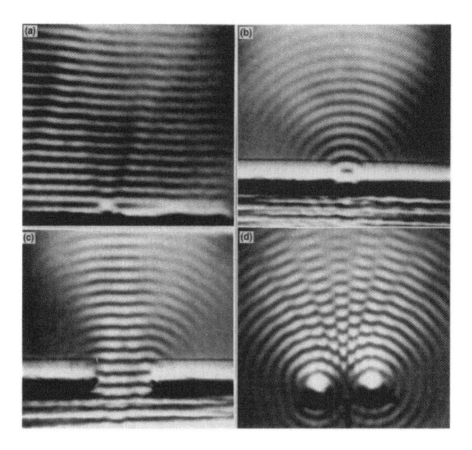

Figure 2.4:   A series of ripple tank photographs of waves generated by vibrating dippers on the surface of water, which behave in a similar manner to light waves.

   (a) A series of plane parallel uninterrupted wavefronts. (b) Plane parallel waves passing through a narrow slit and giving rise to circular wavefronts. (c) Plane parallel waves passing through a wide slit, showing the divergence of the waves at the edges of the slit. (d) Two circular wavefronts (generated at the bottom of the picture by two dippers acting in unison) causing interference as they interact.

light *in vacuo* to that in the medium; for the majority of media its value lies between 1 and 2. The RI is constant for any one medium, but differs according to the wavelength of the light. Some exceptional materials, such as special optical glasses, gemstones and diamond may exceed this higher value. The value of the refractive index for air may be taken as 1. It should be remembered that the refractive index for any medium is *inversely* proportional to the velocity of light in that medium.

   Two familiar examples of the effects of refraction illustrate its importance in microscopical imaging. The 'bent' appearance of a partially-submerged stick, seen at the interface between air and water, is an indication that light has changed direction on passing from one medium to another. Paper, some woven fabrics, and also ground glass, become more transpar-

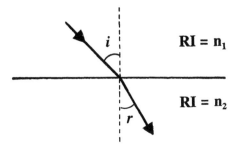

Figure 2.5: Refraction of light.
A diagram to show the refraction of a beam of light travelling in a medium of refractive index n_1 on entering a medium of differing refractive index n_2. The angles of incidence and refraction are indicated by the letters i and r, respectively. According to Snell's Law $sin\ i/sin\ r = n_2/n_1$.

ent when wet, and the closer the RI of the medium is to that of the fluid with which they are wetted, the more transparent they become. This is because light is no longer deviated by the multitude of object/air interfaces, but passes essentially undeviated between object and fluid; this explains the phenomenon of 'clearing' of specimens, and indicates the importance of matching the RI of the mounting medium to that of the specimen.

Light rays typically may be thought of as waves vibrating in all planes perpendicular to the direction of propagation. *Figure 2.6a* shows a beam of unpolarized or natural light coming towards the observer out of the plane of the paper. Four waves have been drawn vibrating at 45° to each other but, of course, in reality all azimuths would be present. If we now constrain the natural light, by some means, so that vibration in only one plane is possible (see *Figure 2.6b*) then we have 'plane-polarized light'. The state of polarization of a beam of light is not immediately apparent,

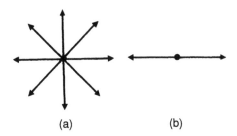

(a)   (b)

Figure 2.6: Natural and plane-polarized light.
Diagram (a) shows beams of unpolarized, natural light emerging from the plane of the paper and travelling towards the observer. Only four waves have been drawn (indicated by lines terminating in arrowheads) although in reality light waves would be present in all azimuths. Diagram (b) shows plane-polarized light in which the vibration directions have been constrained into one plane, here shown as the horizontal.

but it may be recognized if the polarized beam reacts with some other object or medium to produce changes which depend upon the state of polarization of the light. Many transparent substances (e.g. glass and crystals with cubic symmetry) have no such effect and are termed 'isotropic'; light passing through them obeys all the laws of reflection and refraction. Other types of crystal, however, affect light passing through them and are termed 'anisotropic'; the direction of propagation of light passing through them affects their optical properties. Because of the regular arrangement of the molecules, light vibrating in different directions passes through the crystal at different speeds; in other words the crystal has two refractive indices, in directions perpendicular one to the other, and is thus said to be *birefringent* (doubly-refracting). Natural light entering the crystal in most directions becomes polarized into two waves vibrating at right angles. One of these waves behaves normally (the 'ordinary ray'), the other does not, and is thus called the 'extraordinary ray'. Using suitable optical arrangements, it is possible to cause polarized light passing through an anisotropic medium to result in interference and so produce contrasty, often beautifully coloured, images. This topic is considered further in Chapter 5.

2.5 Phase change

A completely transparent object mounted in a medium of different refractive index (or, equally, transparent features *inside* a transparent object) will not affect the amplitude of the light passing through it. There may be some diffraction or scattering at the edges, but the amplitude of such light will normally be so low as to be insignificant with respect to the much brighter direct light passing through the object. If the object is isotropic, the object will not affect the plane of polarization of the incident light. It will, however, change the phase of light which passes through it with respect to that of the light which passes around the object and through the medium alone. For this to occur it is essential that there be a difference in refractive index between the object and its surroundings (or between the various components inside the object itself). This alteration in the phase relationships of the light waves passing through occurs because their speed depends upon the refractive index of the medium through which they are travelling (see *Figure 2.7*). Transparent objects made up of components of different RI are often termed *phase objects*, and they have little, or no, visibility until they are transformed by some optical, or other, technique into amplitude objects.

One method of achieving this transformation was discovered by Frits Zernike when, in the 1930s, he introduced what is now called 'phase-contrast' microscopy. In this technique (see Chapter 6) a very simple manipulation introduces an extra difference of phase between the direct light and the light diffracted by the features of the object, such that summation

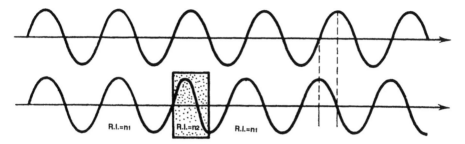

Figure 2.7: Phase change.
A diagram of two beams travelling from left to right in a medium of RI= *n1*. The lower beam passes through a transparent object of a different RI (*n2*) and this causes a change in the phase relationship of this beam with respect to that which does not pass through the object. The amount of this phase change is usually expressed either as a fraction of a wavelength, or as a part of one cycle of 360 degrees. Here a retardation of one quarter of a wavelength, or 90 degrees, is indicated by the distance between the two dotted lines.

of these waves results in a diminution of the amplitude of the resultant (see *Figure 6.2*). This destructive interference occuring in the image causes the transparent phase object to act as if it were an amplitude object and hence appear with the required contrast.

2.6   Fluorescence

When light incident upon matter is absorbed, the molecules of the matter have their electron energy levels increased. There are certain clearly defined energy levels for an electron within an atom, ranging from the ground state through successive excited states S*1, S*2 and so on (see *Figure 2.8*). The higher states differ by progressively smaller amounts of energy until at some limiting value the electron may escape from the atom altogether. When a molecule has absorbed light energy in the form of a photon, it must get rid of this excess energy in some way. Most of this energy is lost by radiation in the form of phosphorescence or fluorescence. The process of absorption and the raising of the energy level of an electron is extremely rapid (in the order of 10^{-13} sec). If the re-radiation or emission occurs 'immediately' (i.e. within about 10^{-9} sec) then the process is called *fluorescence*. If the time between absorption and emission is slow (from about 10^{-4} sec to several seconds) then we speak of *phosphorescence*. It is a characteristic of fluorescence that energy must be supplied to the specimen in the form of short-wave radiation, and that the emitted radiation is in the form of light of a longer wavelength. This light emission makes the specimen truly self-luminous, and if the surplus exciting radiation can be removed, this property of self-luminance allows a tremendous enhancement of contrast to be achieved in the final microscope image.

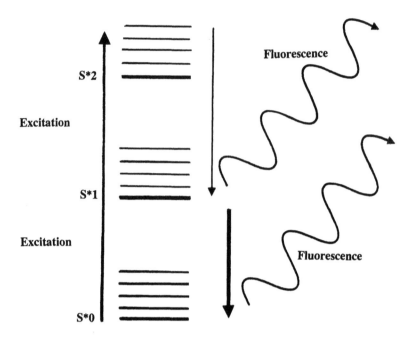

Figure 2.8: Diagram representing three energy states of an atom.
S*0 is the unexcited or ground state, whilst excitation by absorbed incident radiation moves the atom to progressively higher levels of excitation (S*1 and S*2). The process of relaxation occurs spontaneously and the energy absorbed is released as radiation (usually of longer wavelength than the exciting radiation) known as phosphorescence or fluorescence.

Although fluorescence is now one of the most valuable methods of introducing specific contrast into specimens, especially for study with the confocal microscope, it will not be considered in great detail here because it forms the subject of a separate Handbook in this series.

2.7 Stray light

It is worth reminding the reader that although many of the optical effects listed above can enhance contrast, another factor, namely stray light, sometimes called 'glare', may *diminish* contrast. Stray light refers to any light arriving at the image which is not part of the image itself. In some cases the effects are relatively unimportant, but there are instances (e.g. the examination of some ceramic surfaces and many crystals) where it can become of major importance. Stray light originates from multiple unwanted interactions of light with the glass and mechanical parts of a microscope system. These are listed and considered in detail in Chapter 3 and in articles by Dempster (1944), White (1979) and Dodge and White (1980). Attention to the factors causing stray light can significantly improve the quality of the microscope image, and the full and clear discussions provided by Dempster and White are commended to all microscopists.

References

Dempster WT. (1944) Principles of microscopic illumination and the problems of glare. *J. Opt. Soc. Am.* **34**, 695–710.

Dodge AV, White GW. (1980) Further observations on glare in transmitted light microscopy. *Microscopy* **34/1**, 25–46.

Ploem JS. (1995) Reflection-contrast microscopy: an overview. *Proc. R. Microsc. Soc.* **30/3**, 185–192.

Ploem JS, Tanke HJ. (1987) *Introduction to Fluorescence Microscopy* (RMS Handbook no. 10). Oxford University Press, Oxford.

Slayter EM. (1970) *Optical Methods in Biology*. Wiley Interscience, New York.

White GW. (1979) Glare and contrast in the microscope. *Microscopy* **33**, 515–535.

3 Bright-field and Dark-ground Techniques

Specimens for microscopy can broadly be divided into those which are transparent and those which are opaque. A transparent specimen is generally illuminated from the opposite side to the objective (from beneath in a conventional, upright microscope), a situation known as transmitted-light illumination (or trans-illumination). Opaque specimens are illuminated from the same side as the objective, conventionally from above, by epi-illumination (*epi* is Greek for upon or over). In both cases the imaging modes can be divided into bright field or dark field (in light microscopy more usually called dark ground, the term used subsequently in this chapter).

In the case of a transmitting specimen, a featureless, completely empty field would be expected to appear as a uniform disc of light. This is the case in the bright-field image, the most basic of the imaging modes, where the illuminating rays enter the objective lens and 'light up the background'. Features which prevent some of the light from contributing to their corresponding parts of the image will appear darker or coloured, typically by absorption, but also by virtue of other interactions with the illumination.

If the illumination is directed on to a transmitting specimen, from such a direction that it cannot enter the objective lens directly, we have a dark-ground image. A completely featureless, empty area will now appear as a totally dark field, since no light enters the objective. Where light-scattering features are present within the object, these will redirect some of the light so that it enters the objective, and these features will be seen, by virtue of the light which they scatter, bright against a dark background. The Rheinberg illumination technique (see Section 3.7) is a variation of dark ground. *Figure 3.1* shows a schematic representation of bright-field and dark-ground imaging in both transmitted and epi-illumination. A bright-field image results from illumination which falls on to the specimen from *within* the aperture angle of the objective, while illumination from *outside* this angle (either circularly or unilaterally, and shown shaded in the figure) provides a dark-ground image.

In epi-illumination of opaque specimens the equivalent of the featureless, empty glass slide is a surface which acts as a mirror (specimens of metals are generally prepared for observation by polishing to a mirror-like surface). Features of interest may absorb some or all wavelengths; if the surfaces are rough they will reflect like a multitude of mirrors set at

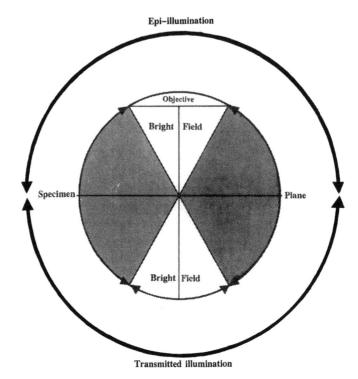

Figure 3.1: A schematic diagram to represent the different imaging modes. Illumination falling on the specimen from above the horizontal specimen plane will give epi-illumination, whilst transmitted light comes from below this plane and passes through the specimen. If the light falls on to the specimen from within the shaded areas in the diagram, that is from outside the acceptance angle of the objective, a dark-ground image will result.

different angles; or they may both absorb and scatter light. In bright-field epi-illumination, light is arranged to fall on to the surface of the specimen through the objective lens (i.e. from *within* the aperture angle of the objective); light-absorbing and light-scattering features will appear dark against the bright mirror-like background. As with trans-illumination, a dark-ground image will result if the illumination arises from *outside* the aperture angle of the objective. In purpose-built instruments the incident light is arranged to pass concentrically around the objective itself, but in many cases (as with a stereomicroscope) unilateral illumination is adequate or even to be preferred.

3.1 Manipulation of the illumination

For general use with amplitude objects (i.e. those stained or naturally-coloured) the illumination is in the form of a full axial cone and achieving contrast is usually not a problem. Transparent objects, on the other hand, illuminated with a full axial cone, generally lack contrast, but if they have an appreciable thickness and are mounted in a medium of different refractive index they will then generate some contrast at their edges. If the edge is parallel to the optic axis of the microscope, the appearance may show very little or no accentuation of the edge (see *Figure 3.2a*); if the edge of the object is curved or markedly inclined to the optic axis then a greater or lesser degree of contrast may be added by refraction of the transmitted light (see *Figure 3.2b*). The intensity of the contrast thus generated will, to a large extent, depend on the difference between the refractive indices of the mountant and of the object.

All teachers who use the microscope in their classes will have noticed the tendency of the students to focus the object and then close the illuminating aperture diaphragm in the condenser so that the objective is working at a fraction of its rated numerical aperture. This, they mistakenly think, gives them a 'better' image. Many students (and even more experienced workers!) take a great deal of convincing that using the full numerical aperture of the objective actually produces a better image! Restricting the working aperture of the condenser-objective system can, however, (if properly used) be of value in helping to obtain a more contrasty image of a transparent object. This increase in contrast is largely produced by the prominent diffraction halo which is formed around the outline of the object. It must be remembered that reducing the numerical aperture in this way will adversely affect the resolution; but if the object is scarcely visible under correct full-cone illumination, then there is little to lose and a controlled use of the aperture diaphragm in this way is admissible. When using axial epi-illumination, reducing the size of the illuminated field diaphragm will significantly improve the contrast in the image, especially when the surface is diffusively reflective and the specimen somewhat trans-

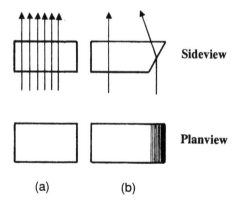

(a)   (b)

Figure 3.2: Light deviation.
(a) Light transmitted normally through a transparent specimen with parallel edges; there is no significant deviation. (b) Light transmitted through a specimen with inclined edges may well be deviated to give a marked enhancement of the edge.

lucent. The edge of the field diaphragm is of course, visible but should be ignored; the benefits of improved contrast outweigh the loss of field of view.

3.1.1 Oblique light

If the illuminating light is non-axial we then speak of oblique illumination. If the angle of the inclination of the rays is such that the direct light would still be accepted by the objective, then a bright-field image will be formed (see *Figure 3.3*), whereas if the angle of inclination of the oblique rays is such that none of the direct light is accepted, then a dark-ground image will result (see Section 3.7). The same criteria apply for epi-illumination (see *Figure 3.4*), although the means by which the obliquity of the light is achieved in practice is usually different.

Oblique light which falls inside the acceptance angle of the objective is often termed internal oblique illumination, whilst that which falls outside the acceptance angle (giving dark ground), would be called external oblique. In both cases, the illumination may be directed on to the specimen from all around (often called 'annular' illumination), or from a single axis, when it may be termed 'azimuthal' oblique light. This latter technique has been used for a very long time but its principal use at the end of the last century was for increasing visibility of fine detail in transparent objects, such as diatom frustules. Interested readers will find a full discussion and illustrations of this in Spitta (1920). Azimuthal oblique transmitted illumination (considered further in Chapter 4) results in an asymmetrically-shaded image of the object and this property is sometimes used as an alternative to the Becke line test to determine whether the refractive index of an object is higher or lower than that of the medium in which it is mounted (Wright, 1913; Robinson and Bradbury, 1992). If the object is mounted in a medium of lower refractive index the shading will appear on the side opposite to that from which the light is entering and vice versa. A full account of this 'half-shadow' method will be found in Mason (1983).

One special use of oblique illumination for the examination of metals is discussed in Gifkins (1970). This method, which he terms 'light cut microscopy', involves shining a very narrow slit-like beam of light at an angle of 45° to a metal surface; the reflected light is imaged by a microscope arranged on the opposite side at a similar angle. The result is an image of the profile of the surface only, the rest being in darkness, which may make the resultant image difficult to interpret. This has been circumvented by a modification, proposed by Tolansky, in which the shadow of a very fine wire is projected on to the surface. The distortions of the shadow, when imaged by the oblique microscope, provide a profile of the irregularities on the surface under study.

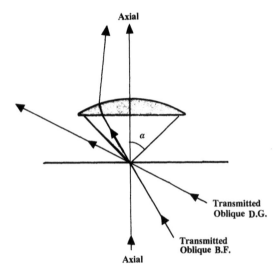

Figure 3.3: A diagram to illustrate transmitted light.

If the light is directed from one side, but at an angle which falls within the acceptance angle of the objective, we have oblique bright-field conditions. If the oblique light is so oblique that it cannot enter the objective then a dark-ground image results. α represents half the acceptance angle of the objective.

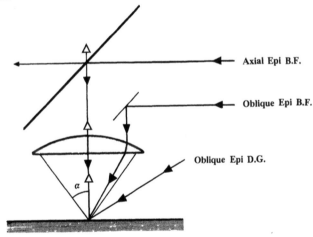

Figure 3.4: Conditions for axial epi-bright-field, oblique epi-bright-field and oblique epi-dark-ground illumination.

(i) Axial epi-bright-field illumination - the line inclined at 45 degrees to the optical axis represents a semi-reflecting mirror surface or dichroic reflector. (ii) In oblique epi-bright field the illumination is reflected on to the specimen by (usually) a small 45 degree prism mounted at the edge of the objective. (iii) Light for oblique epi-dark ground may be shone directly on to the specimen (e.g. from a fibre optic or other source) or it may be reflected on to it at a very oblique angle by means of an annular mirror/lens arrangement surrounding the actual objective. Note that for simplicity, only one imaging ray, on the optical axis, has been drawn. In reality imaging rays will propagate in all directions.

3.2 Polishing, etching and other surface treatments

When opaque materials are to be examined with epi-illumination, the value of staining is much reduced. Some applications are recorded where the voids or cracks in the material have been impregnated with a dye, often fluorescent, to allow their easy visualization and quantitation. In the majority of cases where the surface of the material is naturally smooth and reflective, or where it has been ground and polished, direct epi-illumination techniques of microscopy reveal very little detail. Matters may often be improved by changing the illumination (see Section 3.5). It is also possible to gain contrast by either etching the polished surface or by metallizing it. Etching is commonly used with metal surfaces. Several techniques for etching exist but perhaps the most common is chemical attack. Here the surface of the metal is treated with a chemical which differentially dissolves the various constituents. Strong acids, such as nitric or chromic, may be used, as well as organic acids, like citric and oxalic; suitable etchants are detailed in Haynes (1984). Apart from the introduction of surface relief by the traditional etching methods, techniques exist whereby contrast may be added by the introduction of a gradation or differentiation in surface colour. A controlled chemical oxidation, or the formation of a sulphide on the surface of some components, would be examples of this approach. Other techniques for surface etching involve heating in controlled atmospheres or making the specimen serve as the cathode in a discharge tube system and bombarding it with ions of a gas, such as argon, introduced at reduced pressure into the chamber. Metallization, or 'sputtering', involves the vacuum deposition of a thin film of a reflective metal, such as aluminium or gold, on to the surface of the specimen. It is commonly used in the examination of the surface of polymers and ceramics (Hemsley, 1984). Some use has been made of surface coating of specimens with aluminium to enhance contrast of diatoms by increasing their reflectance when studied with epi-illumination. It is claimed that observation by this technique will allow the resolution of surface structures which are close to the resolving power of the light microscope.

3.3 Enhancing contrast by use of colour – natural colour, staining and illumination changes

In an ideal world, all specimens intended for microscopical observation would be thin, amplitude objects with a strong natural colour. Individual regions of interest within such specimens would be clearly recognizable by a difference in colour or in intensity. It would then be simply a matter of mounting the object and proceeding directly with the examination. This, however, is seldom the case! Naturally coloured objects suitable for direct examination do exist, but they may be too intensely coloured for the light to pass through them or there may be no internal differentiation of detail. These specimens should be examined by reflected light (epi-illumination). For example, in food microscopy, tea leaves or frozen-dried coffee granules are themselves very strongly coloured and appear opaque when mounted. In such cases the problem is not one of adding contrast but exactly the reverse, namely, reducing the absorption of light by the object, either by bleaching the specimen and/or making it transparent before studying it. The same process may be required when biologists are faced with the need to study sections of animal material which has been fixed in fluids containing osmium tetroxide; this procedure leaves a black deposit of lower oxides of osmium in the tissues which must be removed before examination. Suitable agents and the detailed techniques for performing such bleaching are listed in the handbooks devoted to methods of specimen preparation (e.g. Gray, 1954).

Most living biological specimens are virtually transparent, and this often remains after killing and fixation, especially when they have been sliced into thin sections. Traditionally, contrast has been added to such sections by treating them with natural or synthetic dyes, a process called 'staining'. Many hundreds of different dyes have been used for this purpose, some of which are much more effective than others. A complete technology has grown up to produce ever more colourful preparations, and recipe books for staining abound (see, for example, Sanderson, 1994). The end result is to produce from a transparent phase object an amplitude object, in which some, or all, of the transmitted light is absorbed differentially. Consequently, the observer is able to build up a picture of the micro-anatomy of the specimen. The techniques of staining (where there may be little chemical specificity) have been extended into the discipline of 'histochemistry', where a given colour represents the presence and location of a given chemical substance. A specific chemical reaction is carried out on the specimen, already mounted on the slide. When viewed under the microscope the visible, coloured end-product marks the sites where the target substance is to be found. Such techniques will not be further considered here (see, for example, Horobin, 1988; Kiernan, 1990; Pearse, 1972).

Comparable to the use of chemical reactions to locate specific substances is the increasing use of extrinsic markers applied to the specimen, either before or after it has been killed. For example an insoluble finely-ground and suspended pigment, such as carbon, may be injected into an animal, either into the body cavity or into the blood stream. After some time the pigment will have been taken up and stored by the mononuclear phagocytic cells which are located in many sites throughout the body. If the animal is now killed and tissue prepared for microscopical examination it will be possible to locate the active cells of the phagocytic system by their content of the pigment. Such marker techniques are becoming of great importance in biological microscopy, especially with the increasing use of fluorescent-labelled monoclonal antibodies for cell components such as actin, myosin and tubulin. The importance of fluorescent-labelled antibodies for contrast enhancement lies in their complete biological specificity. As their label is fluorescent, all the advantages of this sensitive technique are exploited to the full, especially when allied to the use of confocal microscopy. Immunocytochemical reactions in which the reaction product is localized by means of particles of colloidal gold, especially when ultra-thin sections are in use, are especially suited for study by the reflection contrast microscope technique of Ploem, referred to in Chapter 2.

Contrast may be changed (usually enhanced, but it may be reduced) by alterations in the colour of the light falling on or passing through the specimen. The use of monochromatic light, usually green, is well known in order to minimize chromatic and spherical aberrations in standard achromatic objectives and when phase contrast is used to examine transparent objects. In addition, the wavelength of green light (about 550 nm) lies in the range of greatest sensitivity of the human eye. For maximal resolution of fine detail, slight improvement might be gained by using shorter wavelengths in the blue region, but then the eye loses much of its sensitivity and the detail is far harder to perceive. For black and white photography, however, using blue light may have much to commend it, since many of the films in use are maximally sensitive in this region of the spectrum. In this connection, the possible colour of the mountant should be considered, since this may affect the rendering in a photograph. The most common problem is found with old preparations mounted in Canada balsam, where a marked yellowing of the resin may have taken place with age. A similar problem may be experienced with some high refractive index mountants (e.g. Realgar) formerly used for maximal resolution studies on diatom frustules. If these are photographed with blue light, the mountant may appear completely opaque in the photograph. The fact that an object and its mounting medium may have different transparencies to light of different wavelengths can, on occasion, be used to provide the required contrast. Chitin, for example, although appearing heavily coloured in white light is almost transparent when red or near infra-red illumination is used. Haslam and Hall (1934) give an unusual example of how this principle may be used with ultraviolet light. They were examining lithopone (a compound of zinc sulphide and barium sulphate). The zinc compound is opaque under UV light, whilst the barium salt is transparent in this region of the spectrum. They mounted the lithopone in cumar gum, which has a transparency in UV light intermediate between the zinc and the barium compounds. The resultant micrographs showed the zinc component as black, the barium sulphate as white, whilst the intermediate absorption of the mountant appeared grey.

Colour may also be generated optically in the image. When birefringent specimens are examined between crossed polars, perhaps with the addition of a first-order red plate, colours may result from interference effects. In this case, colour serves not only to improve contrast, but also to give information about the sign and magnitude of the birefringence. An explanation of the way in which such colours arise will be found in Robinson and Bradbury (1992). Similar colours may also be generated when differential interference microscopy (DIC) is used; here the colours emphasize small variations in the optical path difference between areas of the specimen, thereby making any small structural differences very obvious. With phase-contrast microscopy, on the other hand, differences in the object appear only as slight differences in shades of grey, to which our eyes are not very sensitive. Rheinberg illumination, a variant of dark ground, provides images in different colours for background and specimen, with strong contrast and visual appeal (see Section 3.7).

3.4 Colour filters

One very common use of specific wavelength illumination, obtained by introducing colour filters into the light path, is to accentuate or decrease the contrast of a specimen which is either naturally coloured or which has been stained. The general principle is that using a filter of a colour complementary to that of the object will enhance the contrast, whilst using a filter of the same, or a similar colour, will diminish the contrast of the object. Colours are often represented sequentially on a diagram, known as a 'colour circle', in which complementary colours lie diametrically opposite to each other (*see Figure 3.5*). With this diagram it is easy to deter-

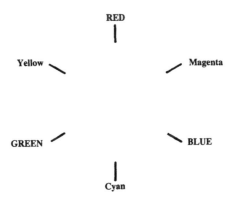

Figure 3.5: The colour circle.
    The three primary colours are printed in capital letters and their complementary, secondary colours shown opposite each of them, in lower case. A filter of the complementary colour will enhance the contrast of objects in the corresponding primary colour.

mine which colour is needed to accentuate the contrast of a given colour. With red-stained specimens, observation in blue/green (cyan) light increases contrast, while red light reduces the effect of the red stain and enables detail in other colours to be seen (see Bradbury, 1985, for further details on the use of filters). Using a longer wavelength will, of course, decrease the resolution of the image. Similarly, an object stained blue would have its contrast increased by the use of its complementary colour, namely yellow, and show the maximum transparency with blue/green light.

3.5 Dark-ground imaging for transmitted light

It is probable that dark-ground imaging has been used from the very earliest days of microscopy (Martin, 1988). Antony van Leeuwenhoek, in a letter to the Royal Society dated 22 January 1675, wrote (translation in Dobell, 1932) "I can demonstrate to myself the globules of blood as sharp and clean as one can distinguish with one's own eyes, without any help of glasses, sand grains that one might bestrew upon a piece of black taffety silk". Although Leeuwenhoek gave no practical details about how this result had been achieved, his description is clearly one of a dark-ground image.

When using non-axial light, the obliquity of the rays with respect to the optical axis might be such that all the direct light passes outside the acceptance angle of the objective. In this situation, if there were no specimen in the optical path, the field of view of the microscope would be absolutely black. If an object is inserted, however, it will diffract and scatter light and such rays will be accepted and form an image. This image will differ from a typical absorption image in that it will be of reversed contrast; that is, the object itself will appear bright on a completely dark background. In dark-ground microscopy the illuminating rays are usually symmetrical with respect to the optical axis, rather than occupying a single azimuth, as with traditional oblique illumination. This means that the light from the condenser forms a hollow cone.

For low-power objectives (in this case meaning those with a numerical aperture below about 0.6), hollow-cone illumination is easily achieved with a conventional condenser fitted with a central opaque stop in its front focal plane and focused so that the apex of the cone of light coincides with the plane of the specimen (*see Figure 3.6*). Such central stops are known as 'patch stops' and may be bought or constructed by the user to suit a particular objective. As the diameter of the stop required depends upon the numerical aperture (NA) of the objective, it is obvious that different objectives will require different sizes for the central opaque disc. Details

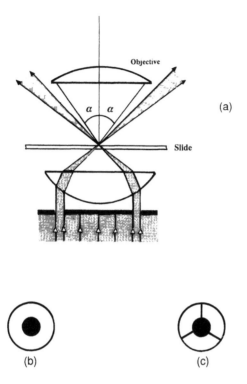

Figure 3.6 : Patch stops.
(a) A diagram of the method of producing transmitted-light dark ground by means of a patch stop in the lower focal plane of the condenser; 2α is the acceptance angle of the objective. Glass and metal patch stops are shown at (b) and (c), respectively.

of the method for determining the size and constructing the stops will be found in Bradbury (1980). With most modern microscopes it is not possible to place the stop in the front focal plane of the condenser as this is not accessible (and, indeed, it should already contain the illuminating aperture iris), but insertion immediately beneath the condenser is usually sufficiently close to the focal plane to give satisfactory dark ground. If a phase-contrast condenser is in use, this will contain several annular stops, one of which may well be of a suitable size to produce acceptable dark ground with the low-power objectives. The use of such a stop has the advantage that it is fitted in the correct conjugate plane and can usually be centred by means of adjustment screws.

If objectives of higher numerical aperture than about 0.6 are intended for use with dark ground, it is usually necessary to use a specialized condenser, rather than insert a patch stop into a standard bright-field condenser. Dark-ground condensers for use with objectives of high aperture are of the reflecting type and it is essential that these condensers are:

(a) accurately centred to the optical axis of the microscope,
(b) in immersion contact with the undersurface of the slide.

The traditional type of reflecting dark-ground condenser is called a 'paraboloid', because it has a single reflecting surface worked in the form of a truncated paraboloid (*see Figure 3.7a*) with a central, axial occluded area. In use, the object is placed at the focus of the hollow cone of light, which has a numerical aperture of 0.9–1.0.

Another type of dark-ground condenser used with transmitted light is called a 'cardioid' and has two mirror surfaces. The first of these is spherical, but the second has the form of a heart-shaped figure, known as a cardioid (*see Figure 3.7b*). Such a system is aplanatic and achromatic but, as with the paraboloid, requires the specimen to be mounted on a slide of the correct thickness, so that the specimen is located at the exact focal point of the hollow cone of rays. As with all high-power dark-ground condensers, the cardioid requires oiling to the undersurface of the slide, thereby making the optical medium homogeneous. The cardioid condenser will deliver an aplanatic hollow cone of light, of NA c. 1.0 to 1.2, therefore, if the objective in use possesses a higher numerical aperture than this, its NA must be reduced in order to get a dark background. Formerly, this was done by fitting a funnel-shaped stop (*see Figure 3.7c*) *inside* the immersion objective. Each objective had its own custom-made funnel stop and no variation in the degree of reduction of the numerical aperture was possible. Funnel stops are now obsolete and objectives intended for high-power dark-ground use are fitted with an integral iris diaphragm, enabling their NA to be reduced progressively, until the optimum result is achieved. All of the current dark-ground reflecting condensers require the specimen to be placed at the focus of the hollow cone of rays. If the slide is too thin (e.g. a 1 mm slide used with a condenser intended to work with slides of 1.5 mm in thickness), there will be difficulty in maintaining the oil film between the upper surface of the condenser and the underside of the slide. To surmount this problem (admittedly, now much less important than before the days of standardized thickness slides), some dark-ground condensers have been designed with variable focus.

Formerly, in fluorescence microscopy with transmitted light, where a very wide angle cone of short wave blue or UV light was used to illuminate the specimen, dark-ground condensers were often used. This was in order to minimize excess transmitted exciting radiation entering the objective, along with the longer wavelength fluorescence emitted by the specimen. With fluorescence microscopy, epi-illumination has great advantages as alignment problems are minimized (since the same lens serves as both condenser and objective). There is also the advantage that an easy change-over between the fluorescence dark ground and transmitted light can be made, or a separate type of contrast technique, such as phase contrast, may be used in the transmitted light mode at the same time as the epi-fluorescence.

With dark ground, no direct light enters the objective; intense light sources must, therefore, be used. Modern light sources, such as tungsten-halogen bulbs, ensure that this is not so much of a problem as it was in the

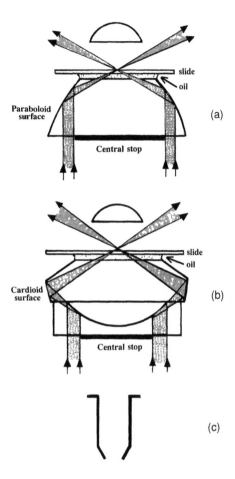

Figure 3.7: Paraboloid and cardioid condensers.
(a) A sectional diagram of a paraboloid reflecting condenser used for high-power dark ground. It is usually solid glass with a central stop fixed to the lower surface and must be used in immersion contact with the underside of the slide. (b) A diagrammatic section of a cardioid condenser. The light is reflected twice, once from a convex spherical surface, and again from the inner aspect of a cardioid surface. As with the paraboloid, this type of condenser is immersed to the slide. (c) A section of a 'funnel stop' used in older high-aperture objectives to reduce their numerical aperture sufficiently for a satisfactory dark-ground image to be obtained.

early days of dark-ground imaging. As all the condensers used for transmitted dark ground have some form of central occlusion of the light, it is important to note that the illuminating aperture diaphragm *must* be fully open; failure to observe this is the most common cause of unsatisfactory dark-ground images.

Dark ground, like phase contrast (considered later in Chapter 6), does not work well with strongly coloured specimens. It does provide good images of poorly-stained or transparent objects, however, in which the details appear bright against a dark background. Red blood cells or small glass spheres (often known as 'ballotini'; *see Figure 3.8*), for example, appear with bright contours outlining their edges. With this type of illumination, which provides extreme contrast at the edges of objects, it is important to ensure that the slides, covers and the mountant are as clean

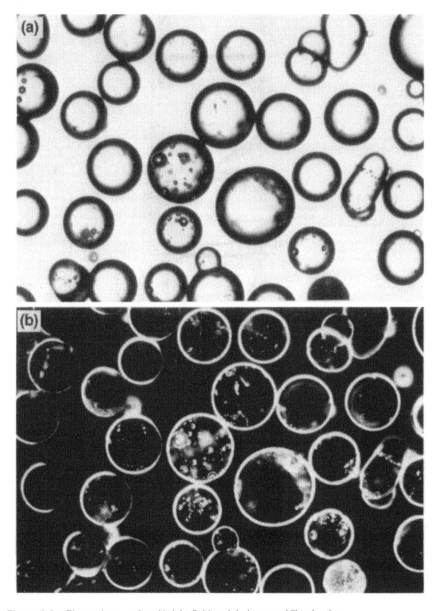

Figure 3.8: Photomicrographs of bright-field and dark-ground illumination.
(a) Photomicrograph of small glass spheres (ballotini), mounted in water and seen with bright-field illumination; the ballotini are outlined very strongly because of the difference in refractive indices of object and mountant. (b) The same field with dark-ground illumination; contrast is now reversed with respect to (a).

as possible, otherwise small dirt particles or scratches (which also diffract and scatter light) can seriously degrade the quality of the image or micrograph.

The use of dark ground as a contrast technique enables the observation of many fine details which are not seen with conventional bright-field microscopy because of the lack of contrast in the specimen. Barer (1955) comments, with respect to dark-ground illumination that, "In the form most frequently used, i.e., oblique dark ground illumination, in which the object is illuminated by rays of an obliquity greater than can be accepted by the microscope objective, there is an asymmetrical interception of light diffracted by the object which results in great exaggeration of edges and discontinuities."

It is this, together with the fact that the object appears as self-luminous on a dark background, that gives the impression that the actual resolution is increased. Although the presence of small objects may be more easily *detected*, it cannot be said that any more real detail may be perceived in the image.

Readers familiar with the Abbe experiments, using diffraction gratings and slit or hole diaphragms inserted into the back focal plane of the objective to occlude selectively some of the diffraction maxima, will immediately realise that it is possible to use this approach to obtain dark-ground (reversed contrast) images. If, instead of occluding one or more of the diffraction orders, the central or zero order (which represents the direct light) is blocked off, the image will show bright contrast upon a dark ground. In practice this approach is not much used for standard dark ground, although it is used in one form of dispersion staining as realised by McCrone (see Section 4.2).

3.6 Dark-ground epi-illumination

With bright-field epi-illumination the objective acts as its own condenser, the illuminating direct light entering from 90° to the optical axis into which it is reflected by means of a semi-reflecting mirror, cover slip or small offset prism. Dark ground may be obtained with epi-illumination, but the arrangements for obtaining a hollow cone of annular incident direct light of sufficient obliquity are quite different from those in use with transmitted light; some form of co-axial system is needed. The incident light enters at 90° to the optic axis and is passed around and outside the barrel of the objective, before being reflected around the optic axis by an annular mirror system placed at 45°. The light is concentrated obliquely on to the specimen by a second annular mirror, or lens system, surrounding the objective itself (*see Figure 3.9*). Each objective has its own illuminating lenses, or mirrors, mounted in a metal mount or 'skirt' which may be

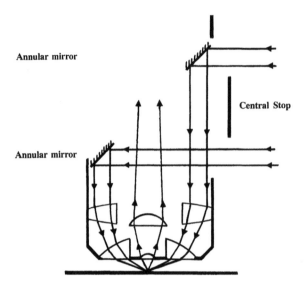

Figure 3.9: Arrangement for dark-ground epi-illumination.
A diagram of the arrangement of annular mirror and lenses surrounding an objective which allows dark-ground with epi-illumination.

adjustable to allow control over the degree of obliquity of the annular illumination.

In some of the large modular research microscopes, such as the Leica DM series, the Olympus BX system and microscopes by Zeiss, the reflected-light dark-ground system is mounted in a separate block which inserts above the nosepiece, a system made easier by the use of infinity-corrected optics in these newer stands. A comparison between the image of part of an integrated circuit seen in epi-bright field (a) and epi-dark ground (b) is shown in *Figure 3.10*.

3.7 Rheinberg illumination

This method of illumination (Rheinberg, 1896) may be regarded simply as a variant of transmitted-light dark ground. It resembles patch stop dark ground in that the effect is achieved by inserting a filter made up of two complementary colours into the front focal plane of the condenser. The central circle is usually the darker colour (often deep blue or green) and this is surrounded by an annulus of the complementary colour (*see Figure 3.11a, b*); occasionally the central area is opaque (*see Figure 3.11c, d, e*). The diameter of the central circular disc is determined by the numerical aperture of the objective in use and will, therefore, differ for different objectives. This means that several filters are needed to allow this type of

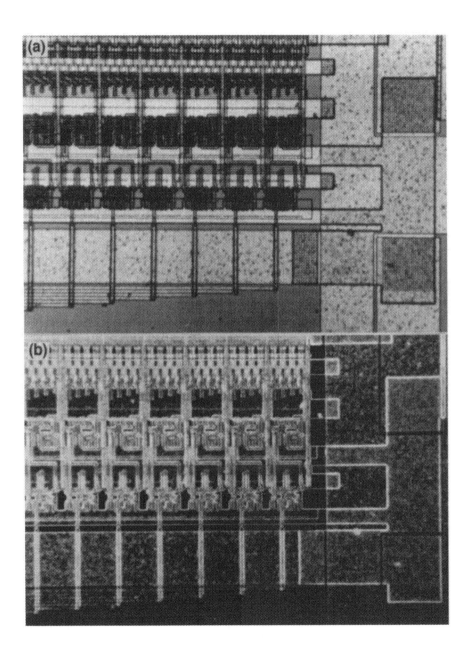

Figure 3.10: Comparison of epi-bright field and epi-dark ground.
    A comparison between the image of part of an integrated circuit seen in epi-bright field (a) and epi-dark ground (b).

illumination to be used with objectives of various apertures. As with standard dark-ground illumination, if Rheinberg is to be used with oil-immersion objectives, then they must have their numerical aperture significantly reduced, either by a funnel stop or by an internal iris diaphragm.

At one time, sets of Rheinberg discs were commercially available, but now workers wishing to use this technique must construct their own discs from gelatine filter material, mounted on some form of carrier. With a standard Rheinberg filter (a central circular stop of one colour, surrounded by an annulus of another colour), scattered light arising from objects illuminated by the annular oblique rays will be accepted by the objective, causing them to appear in that colour, whilst the background will appear in the colour of the central stop. This is because the direct light passing through the annular area of the filter is too oblique to fall within the acceptance angle of the objective. It should be noted, however, that because the central stop is *not* opaque, the objective will accept direct light of this colour.

In addition to the annular stops, Rheinberg also designed a bi-sector stop and a quadrant stop (see *Figure 3.11c,d*). These are used when the specimen on the stage has a definite orientation. For example, the warp and the weft of a fabric may be shown in two different colours against either a completely black background or one of a third, darker colour. Rheinberg illumination may not give any more information about the specimen, but it does produce images of striking beauty! This means that it has found favour with illustrators, and to some extent with workers in the field of textiles, crystals, Foraminifera and similar aquatic organisms, and is frequently used to create spectacular images for displays. The construction of Rheinberg stops is detailed in Bradbury (1980).

Taylor (1984) published a variant on the classical Rheinberg procedure which he calls 'spectral Rheinberg'. He comments that, "All bright field contrast enhanced images must consist of (a) the background rays (b) the refracted rays and (c) the diffracted rays. Dark-ground methods easily separate the background and diffracted rays, but the vital refracted rays that are bent in passing through the specimen are deviated by such a small angle from the background rays that most of them are lost, the image being composed mainly of those rays that are scattered by the more strongly refracting material and therefore not giving information about weakly refractile specimens that is needed for the most informative images. Phase and anoptral contrast effectively separate these rays to yield a very complete image that is basically bright field and well contrasted."

In the front focal plane of the condenser Taylor places a stop with a central opaque spot. This spot is roughly equal in diameter to the opening in the illuminating aperture iris when this is set for optimum contrast for the objective in use. The spot is surrounded by a coloured annulus which, in turn, is surrounded by a clear outer zone (see *Figure 3.11e*). He claims that this system removes the inherent glare which may be troublesome with traditional Rheinberg illumination.

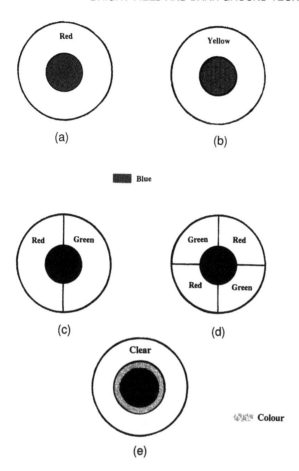

Figure 3.11: Diagrams of various forms of Rheinberg illumination stops.
Diagram (a) and (b) have deep blue central spots and are surrounded by red and yellow outers, respectively. The background from using these would be deep blue and the scattered light from the objects would be either red or yellow. (c) An opaque central stop with a bisector red/green surround. (d) A quadrant stop which will colour scattering objects orientated in different azimuths red or green. (e) This is the type of stop used for Taylor's 'spectral Rheinberg', as described in the text.

Two other methods of providing two-colour contrast may be mentioned briefly. One, (MacConaill, 1955), uses light of one colour (usually green) for trans-illumination, whilst the opaque specimen is illuminated from *above* with light of the complementary colour. This technique requires a very careful balancing of the intensities of both light sources in order to achieve success.

Another colour contrast method, specifically intended for diatoms, was introduced by Wilson (1966). He fitted an opaque disc which had an off-centre hole in the front focal plane of the condenser in order to produce an azimuthal beam of extremely oblique rays of white light which falls outside the acceptance angle of the objective. This would give a dark-ground effect with reversed contrast if any rays were diffracted by an object on the stage; any such diffracted light, was, however, prevented from participating in image formation by a semi-circular stop placed in the back focal plane of the objective. The oblique rays of the direct light were reflected *back* on to the diatoms mounted on the slide by means of a curved mirror fitted to the outside of the objective. They were then diffracted, by the regular periodicity of the frustules, to produce rays which entered the objective and were not occluded by the semicircular stop, so that these rays formed a coloured image of the diatoms on a dark background. Since the colour is formed by diffraction due to the regular periodicity of the frustules, it will differ according to their spacing and, hence, if the same light source is used, different genera of diatoms will show in different colours.

3.8 Stray light

It is worth mentioning that although the optical adjustments listed above can enhance contrast, another factor – namely stray light – can be just as important in reducing contrast. Stray light, sometimes known as 'glare', is a haze of light over the whole image, which diminishes contrast. In some cases the effects are relatively unimportant, but there are instances (e.g. the examination of ceramic surfaces, the examination of many crystals) where stray light can become a major nuisance. Stray light has multiple origins in a microscope system; these are listed and considered in detail in articles by Beck (1922), Dempster (1944) and White (1979). Attention to the factors causing stray light can significantly improve the quality of the microscope image, and the full and clear discussions provided by Dempster and White are recommended to all microscopists. Dempster recognises that stray light may originate in:

- the tube
- the lens mounts
- the lens elements
- the slide and coverslip
- the eye

1. 'Tube glare', as Dempster calls it, is formed by stray light reflected from improperly baffled, and/or blackened, interior surfaces of the microscope tube. It should not constitute much of a problem with the modern instrument .
2. Stray light originating in the lens mount as a result of extreme peripheral rays refracted by the front hemispherical lens element hitting the inside of the lens mount may result from using too large a cone of light

for the NA of the objective in use, or illuminating too large an area of the specimen. The obvious solution is to set the size of the illuminated field diaphragm so that only the area of specimen actually imaged is illuminated and to adjust the aperture diaphragm in the condenser to give a cone of light of about nine tenths of the aperture of the objective.

3. With the advent of multiple coatings on the optical surfaces of the microscope lenses and prisms, 'lenticular glare', which is caused by the reflection of light from air/glass interfaces inside the objective, is minimal and careful control of the illuminated area and of the working aperture will reduce it even further.

4. Dempster's 'slide glare' is caused by light reflected from the undersurface of the slide and from the upper surface of the cover. He recommends controlling this by the use of a homogeneous system, that is, one in which the undersurface of the slide is oiled to the upper lens of the condenser and the coverslip is oiled to the front lens of the objective. Nowadays, the condenser is very seldom oiled to the slide (a practice much used formerly, principally not for control of stray light, but to extract the absolute maximum resolution from the objective). Immersion objectives, on the other hand, are now more commonly used than before, largely because of their increased aperture (and, hence, light gathering power), and their use does help to minimize stray light.

5. Dempster appreciated the fact that extraneous light entering above the ocular from the side (i.e. at the periphery of the field of view of the eye), or being reflected by the upper surface of the ocular itself or spectacles could also cause glare; this he termed 'eye glare', and it can be minimized by careful attention to the illumination of the room.

Dempster maintained that stray light was lowest, and contrast highest, when the aperture diaphragm was closed so that the working aperture of the system was restricted to one third of that of the objective; these conditions he termed 'contrast illumination', as compared with the nine tenths full-cone illumination advocated by many microscopists, which Dempster designated 'controlled' illumination. He regarded an image formed with the NA of the objective reduced below one third as unsatisfactory because of the prominent diffraction bands which then appear to outline the object.

References

Barer R. (1955) Phase-contrast, interference contrast and polarizing microscopy. In *Analytical Cytology* (ed. RC Mellors). McGraw Hill, New York, pp. 169–272.

Beck C. (1922) The illumination of microscopic objects: glare and flooding with transmitted light. *J. R. Microsc. Soc.* **42**, 399–405.

Bradbury S. (1980) Getting the best out of your microscope. *Proc. R. Microsc. Soc.* **15**, 270–279.

Bradbury S. (1985) Filters in microscopy. *Proc. R. Microsc. Soc.* **20**, 83–91.

Dempster WT. (1944) Principles of microscopic illumination and the problems of glare. *J. Opt. Soc. Am.* **34**, 693–710.

Dobell C. (1932) *Antony van Leeuwenhoek and his 'Little Animals'.* Bale & Danielsson, London.

Gifkins RC. (1970) *Optical Microscopy of Metals.* Pitman, London.

Gray P. (1954) *The Microtomist's Formulary and Guide.* Maple Press, New York.

Haslam GS, Hall CH. (1934) Microscopic study of pigments using ultraviolet light. *J. Opt. Soc. Am.* **24**, 14–18.

Haynes R. (1984) *Optical Microscopy of Materials.* International Textbook Co., London.

Hemsley DA. (1984) *The Light Microscopy of Synthetic Polymers* (RMS Handbook no. 7). Oxford University Press, Oxford.

Horobin RW. (1988) *Understanding Histochemistry: Selection, Evaluation and Design of Biological Stains.* Ellis Horwood, Chichester.

Kiernan JA. (1990) *Histological and Histochemical Methods; Theory and Practice* (2nd edn). Pergamon Press, Oxford.

Mason CW. (1983) *Handbook of Chemical Microscopy* (4th edn) Vol. 1. John Wiley & Sons, New York.

MacConaill MA. (1955) Double-illumination microscopy. *Nature* **176**, 877.

Martin LV. (1988) Early history of dark ground illumination with the microscope. *Microscopy* **36**, 124–138.

Pearse AGE. (1972) *Histochemistry: Theoretical and Applied* (3rd edn). Churchill Livingstone, Edinburgh, London.

Rheinberg J. (1896) On an addition to the methods of microscopical research, by a new way of optically producing colour-contrast between an object and its background, or between definite parts of the object itself. *J. R. Microsc. Soc.* **Ser II, XVI**, 373–388.

Robinson PC, Bradbury S. (1992) *Qualitative Polarized-light Microscopy* (RMS Handbook no. 9). Oxford University Press, Oxford.

Sanderson JB. (1994) *Biological Microtechnique* (RMS Handbook no. 28). BIOS Scientific Publishers, Oxford.

Spitta EJ. (1920) *Microscopy: the Construction, Theory and Use of the Microscope* (3rd edn). J. Murray, London.

Taylor RB. (1984) Rheinberg updated. *Proc. R. Microsc. Soc.* **19**, 253–256.

White GW. (1979) Glare and contrast in the microscope. *Microscopy* **33**, 515–535.

Wilson SD. (1966) A reflection-diffraction microscope for observing diatoms in color. *Appl. Optics* **5**, 1683–1684.

Wright FE. (1913) Oblique illumination in petrographic microscopic work. *Am. J. Sci.* **35**, 63–82.

4 Refractive Differences between Specimen and Mountant; the 'Becke line'

It is possible to exploit any difference (or lack of it) between the refractive index (RI) of the mountant and a transparent specimen to help in the visualization of that object. The closer the refractive indices of the object and the medium surrounding it become, the less will be the contrast, and if the two indices match, the object may even become invisible unless the working aperture of the system is dramatically reduced. This variation in contrast due to RI differences and aperture has been appreciated for some time; for example, it is referred to, with respect to sand grains mounted in Canada balsam, by Sorby (1877) "If the aperture of both the object glass and condenser is large, and the grains are mounted in Canada balsam, little or no trace of them may be visible, but by reducing the aperture their outline becomes more and more distinct, and the shading greater and greeater, until in certain cases it may become so dark as to obscure certain characters."

The use of variations in the refractive index of the mountant to control contrast has been studied extensively and various workers have described techniques for expressing this in some quantitative way. For example, Dall (1985) introduced the concept of 'visibility index' (defined as the difference between the refractive index of silica and that of the mountant), for use in the high resolution study of siliceous diatom frustules. Dall considered diatom frustules mounted in air, having a visibility index of 0.46, to be easy to see, whilst if they were mounted in Canada balsam this figure dropped to 0.07 and their visibility was much reduced. In contrast, mounting the frustules in Realgar (which has a refractive index of c. 2.45) increased the visibility index to a value of 1.0, enabling the diatoms to be seen more clearly again.

A similarity in refractive indices between an object and its surrounding medium can be exploited, when using plane polarized light alone (i.e. without an analyser), for the study of transparent anisotropic crystals and biological objects, such as holothurian spicules. Such specimens effectively have two refractive indices. If mounted in a medium with a RI identical to one of these they will become virtually invisible, but if the specimen is rotated through 90°, the mismatch in refractive indices will result in a great increase in contrast and hence visibility. A fuller explanation of this phenomenon is given in Robinson and Bradbury (1992).

When there is an edge between two crystals of different refractive index, or between a crystal and its surrounding medium, the edge may be strongly accentuated when a narrow parallel axial or oblique beam of light is used. This phenomenon manifests as a bright line surrounding the edge of the object which, on altering the plane of focus of the microscope, will move towards the area of greatest refractive index (see *Figure 4.1*). This line is called the Becke line and it is usually used in the measurement of refractive index, although it may be of value in helping in some morphological observations.

Wood (1934) has shown that with transparent mineral grains mounted in organic media which differ from them in refractive index, the strongly shadowed edges which result when they are viewed by oblique light are sometimes useful as a means of enhancing contrast. For any substance there is usually a variation in refractive index with the wavelength of the light at which it is measured, a phenomenon which is called 'dispersion'; the 'dispersion curve' is a plot of such variation of refractive index against wavelength. Organic liquids usually have steeper dispersion curves than inorganic solids (see *Figure 4.2*), and if the refractive indices are equal for a wavelength in the middle of the visible spectrum, then the solid grain will usually have a higher refractive index for blue light. If white light is used to illuminate the transparent particle, colour fringes are often produced at its edge, where the light is incident at an angle other than normal (see *Figure 4.3*), the particle tending to converge the red wavelengths and diverge the blue. This is the 'Christiansen effect' (Wright, 1911), whereby the light of the colour for which the RIs are identical will be transmitted unchanged, but that of other colours will be deviated by refraction. The result is a colour fringe of either yellow/orange/red or blue, depending on whether the RI of the liquid is lower or higher than that of the grain. With unilateral oblique light, opposite sides of the particle will appear to show these colours. Dodge (1948) used this phenomenon in his 'dark-field colour immersion method' which he used for measurement of refractive index rather than for contrast generation.

4.1 Dispersion staining

Dispersion staining is an optical technique which uses the Christiansen effect to give colour to transparent substances. In its standard form, dispersion staining was developed by Crossmon (1949) for use with biological sections, although the full potential was realised by McCrone who, in papers published in collaboration with Brown and others (1963; 1978), outlined the theory of the technique and its applications to the study and identification of crystals and fibres. The strong colours of dispersion staining are produced when a transparent object, such as a crystal, is immersed in a liquid with a refractive index very near that of the object and viewed with transmitted white light. For the colours to appear clearly it is essen-

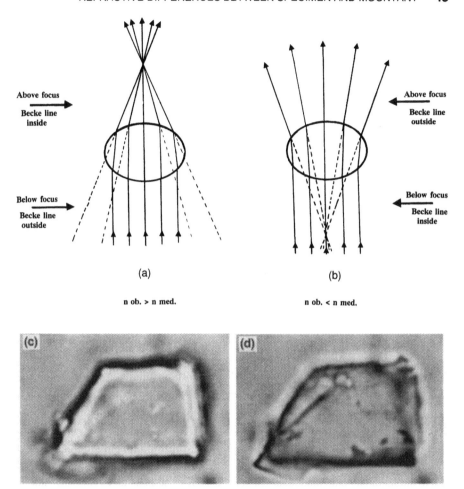

Figure 4.1: A diagram to show the formation of the Becke line.

In (a) the transparent object has a *higher* refractive index than the mountant and on raising the objective above focus the bright Becke line appears inside the object, whilst on moving below focus the Becke line is seen to surround the specimen. (b) Shows that when the specimen has a *lower* refractive index than the mountant, the situation is reversed and on raising the objective above focus the bright Becke line now appears to surround the object. (c) A photomicrograph of crushed salt mounted in oil taken above focus; the Becke line appears *within* the crystal, thus we can deduce that the RI of the crystal is higher than that of the mountant. (d) This micrograph shows the situation below true focus; the Becke line is now *outside* the crystal.

tial that the dispersion curves of solid and immersion liquid should inter-sect sharply at a given wavelength, as shown in *Figure 4.2*. It is easy to calculate the linear deviation of a diffracted ray in the back focal plane of a microscope objective knowing the focal length of the objective and the angular deviation of the ray. This latter depends on the difference in re-fractive indices between the mountant and the particle for any given wave-length. Crossmon and McCrone, and others, have used this to design and

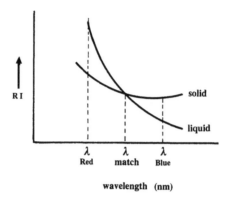

Figure 4.2: A diagram of the so-called 'dispersion curves' for a hypothetical solid and liquid.
This plot of refractive index against wavelength shows that in the red region of the spectrum (λ red) the RI of the liquid is much higher than that of the solid, whereas in the blue (λ blue) the reverse is true. Somewhere between these wavelengths is a point (λ match) at which the RIs of the solid and liquid are equal. At this point the optical contrast of the solid mounted in the liquid will be at a minimum.

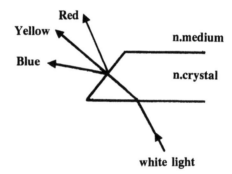

Figure 4.3: The 'Christiansen' effect.
A crystal with a refractive index (n. crystal), mounted in a liquid medium of different refractive index (n. medium), when illuminated with white light at an angle will appear fringed with colour, the red rays being bent in towards the body of the crystal.

place screens in the back focal plane of objectives intended for use with dispersion staining in order to occlude either the rays with approximately zero dispersion or those in which the linear deviation was significantly different from zero. These alternatives are called annular screening and central screening respectively; annular screening uses a disc with a small central hole of c. 2 mm in diameter mounted in the back focal plane so that only the less-deviated rays will be used in image formation (see *Figure 4.4a*). Central screening is done with a centrally-placed opaque stop of about 4 mm in diameter in the back focal plane of the objective (see *Figure 4.4b*). The microscope condenser is usually partially closed, to restrict the aperture of the axial light, in order to achieve correct and brilliant dispersion staining. If it is assumed that the refractive index match of the particle and the medium is correct for the wavelength of the sodium D-line (c. 590 nm), then the centrally placed opaque stop of the central screen will block the unrefracted axial beam and allow white light, *minus* the wavelengths around the sodium D-line, to pass. This will produce an image in which the particles appear with reddish/purple or blue edges on a dark background. Conversely, the annular stop will only allow the wavelengths close to 590 nm to pass and form the image, so this will show particles with yellow edges in bright field. The edge colour seen with the

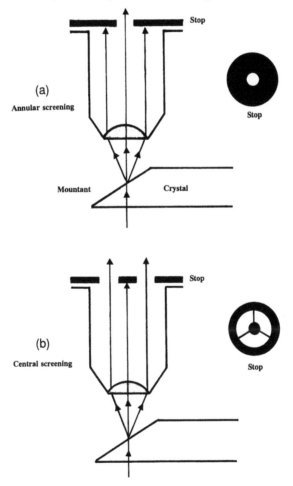

Figure 4.4: Diagrams of the two arrangements used in Crossmon's dispersion staining.
In this system a crystal surface illuminated by white light deviates the red and blue rays of light passing through it. In (a) there is an annular stop with a small central hole fitted in the back focal plane of the objective. The red and blue deviated rays are blocked so the crystal will appear in bright field with an edge coloured by white light minus red and blue (i.e. yellow). In diagram (b) the central stop is in use and the reverse occurs. Undeviated light is stopped off and the image of the crystal appears in dark ground with reddish-purple edges.

two types of stop will be complementary and the contrast with the central screen will resemble that obtained with traditional dark-ground illumination. Special objectives are available for dispersion staining studies with metal stops on a turntable located in the back focal plane of the objective. Full details of the technique are given in the reference by Brown and McCrone (1963) and many examples of its use in the identification of transparent substances are given in Brown *et al.* (1963). An alternative, full-aperture dispersion staining method has been published by Speight (1977).

References

Brown KM, McCrone WC. (1963) Dispersion staining part I – theory, method and apparatus. *The Microscope* **13/11,** 311–322.

Brown KM, McCrone WC, Kuhn R, Forlini L. (1963) Dispersion staining part II – the systematic application to the identification of transparent substances. *The Microscope* **14/2,** 39–54.

Crossmon PC. (1949) The "dispersion staining" method for the selective coloration of tissue. *Stain Technol.* **24,** 61–65.

Dall HE. (1985) Mounting method for high resolution optical microscopy. *Microscopy* **35/4,** 280–284.

Dodge NB. (1948) The dark-field color immersion method. *Am. Mineral.* **33,** 541–549.

McCrone WC. (1978) Dispersion staining colours. *The Microscope* **26,** 109–120.

Robinson PC, Bradbury S. (1992) *Qualitative Polarized Light Microscopy* (RMS Handbook no. 9). Oxford University Press, Oxford.

Sorby HC. (1877) Anniversary address of the President. *Monthly Microsc. J.* **XVIII,** 113–136.

Speight RG. (1977) An alternative dispersion staining technique. *The Microscope* **5,** 215–225.

Wright FE. (1911) Oblique illumination in petrographic microscopic work. *Am. J. Sci.* **35,** 63–82.

Wood RW. (1934) *Physical Optics* (3rd edn). Macmillan, New York.

5 Polarized-light Techniques

As mentioned in Section 2.4, natural light consists of waves vibrating in all planes perpendicular to the direction of propagation. Light vibrating in a single plane can be selected from natural light by passing it through a device known as a 'polar'. This light is then said to be 'plane-polarized'. If a second polar is placed with its permitted vibration perpendicular to that of the first, none of the plane-polarized light will be transmitted through it. In this position the polars are said to be 'crossed'. The essential special components of a polarized-light microscope are two such polars, known respectively as the 'polarizer' and the 'analyser'.

For some substances the velocity (or wavelength) of a beam of light passing through them is constant, whatever the direction of passage: these transparent substances are thus said to be 'isotropic', and include transparent amorphous substances, such as glass and cubic crystals. There are other materials, however, for which this statement does not apply, and which are called 'anisotropic'. Anisotropic materials may include stressed glass and polymers, as well as many types of crystals. When a beam of light passes through an anisotropic material the light is split into two rays which are plane-polarized, that is, they are vibrating in mutually perpendicular planes. For a uniaxial substance (the simplest case) one such ray obeys the normal laws of refraction and has a constant velocity whatever its direction. This is called the ordinary ray. The other ray has a velocity which varies according to its direction in the material and hence it is known as the extraordinary ray. This behaviour is due to some kind of directionality of structural properties of the material and this in turn gives rise to a directional effect in the optical properties of the material. There are thus two refractive indices, one associated with each ray; for a uniaxial substance the refractive index is fixed for the ordinary ray but is variable for the extraordinary ray. The substance is said to show 'double refraction' and the numerical difference between the refractive index values of ordinary and extraordinary rays is called the 'birefringence'. Birefringence may be grouped into four main categories termed 'intrinsic', 'form', 'strain' and 'flow'. Intrinsic birefringence is characteristic of the molecular structure of all anisotropic compounds except cubic crystals, whilst form birefringence results from a regular arrangement of submicroscopic structures held in a medium of different refractive index from themselves. An example of form birefringence is shown by the starch granule in which the molecules of starch have a radial arrangement. If a regular arrangement of structures arises during movement, as in the pseudopodia of a protozoan such as *Amoeba*, then flow birefringence results. If a regular arrangement of particles or molecules is induced by mechanical factors then this may give rise to strain birefringence. This latter is often seen in glass which has been rapidly cooled and hence stressed, or in transparent materials such as plastics under stress. This stress produces directional mechanical changes which alter the optical properties in a directional way. It is for this reason that objectives intended specifically for use with a polarized-light microscope are constructed from strain-free glass.

Double refraction can be detected by its effects on plane-polarized light which is allowed to pass through the doubly refracting object and then has its resulting components recombined by passsage through a second polar with its vibration at right angles to that of the polarizer.

As the plane-polarized components pass through anisotropic materials, the peaks and troughs of the corresponding light waves no longer remain 'in step', since their velocities are different. This difference is expressed as an 'optical path difference', and it also becomes greater as the material becomes thicker. Since the two wave trains arise from the same light source they are coherent, and there is thus the possibility of either constructive or destructive interference leading to contrast enhancement when the two waves leave the material and are recombined.

Polarized-light microscopy is much used in materials science, not only to detect anisotropy, but also to measure and characterize substances by the amount and nature of their birefringence. Biologists, on the other hand, tend not to use polarized light very often. This may perhaps be due to the failure to understand the principles of polarized light which are often expressed in a very mathematical fashion unlikely to appeal to biologists. More likely, however, is the fact that much biological material shows only relatively weak birefringence with poor contrast. Notable exceptions include starch grains, cellulose and crystalline inclusions in plant cells, insect cuticle and sections of bone and striated muscle. A full description of the basic concepts of polarized-light microscopy will be found in Bennet (1950), Galopin and Henry (1972), Mason (1983) and Robinson and Bradbury (1992).

5.1 The polarized-light microscope

Although the measurement of birefringence may be of diagnostic importance, especially in mineralogical microscopy, double refraction or birefringence may also be used as a means of introducing contrast. For this it is usual to use a specially designed polarized-light microscope. A detailed account of the instrument itself, and its accessories, is given in the book by Robinson and Bradbury (1992).

Originally, the polarized-light microscope used Nicol prisms to polarize and analyse the light. The Nicol prism is a rhombohedron of calcite, cut diagonally, ground and polished and cemented together with Canada balsam. It was invented by William Nicol in 1828. 'Polaroid' plastic sheet (invented by Edwin Land in 1932) is now universally used in place of Nicol prisms, allowing the use of much larger condenser and objective apertures. In the case of a microscope using reflected light for the examination of opaque materials, the polarizer is usually placed before the beam splitter which deflects the light into the optical axis of the microscope. As many types of beam-splitting prism have some effect on the degree of polarization of the light, it is desirable that the beam splitter in these instruments be made of plane glass, orientated at 45° to the optical axis. The Smith reflector (described in detail in Hallimond, 1970) is even better, since it causes less depolarization of the light.

Polarized-light microscopes have provision for the rotation in the optical axis of either the polarizer and the analyser, and for their removal from the system. In addition, there is a slot above the objective, and below the analyser, for the insertion of additional optical elements called 'compensators' or retardation plates. These are typically used for the measurement of the degree of birefringence, but one type (the first-order red plate), is often used for the introduction of strong colour contrast. Most microscopes intended primarily for use with polarized light will also be fitted with a rotating stage and a Bertrand lens. This latter, when inserted into the optical path, acts in conjunction with the eyepiece to serve as a telescope, enabling easy inspection of the back focal plane of the objective. The Bertrand lens is primarily used with conoscopic illumination to examine interference figures produced by some crystals as an aid to their identification.

When a microscope is fitted with a polarizer in the light path orientated with its preferred direction East–West (the directions are conventionally described by reference to points of the compass) and an analyser placed further on in the optical system with its preferred vibration directions North–South, no direct light will pass and the microscope field will appear dark. If an unstained, birefringent specimen is now placed on the stage between the polarizer and the analyser there will be, when the specimen is in certain orientations, a resultant beam of light emerging from the specimen which has a component orientated at an angle to the E–W plane of vibration of the polarizer. Hence, this emergent beam will have some components in the N–S direction which will be able to pass through the analyser, making the object appear bright and clearly visible against the dark field of the microscope.

5.2 Observations with a single polar

Within a birefringent material the refractive index varies according to the vibration direction of the light passing through it. When plane-polarized light is used for illumination, without any analyser in the system, it will be found that the contrast of a doubly refracting object increases to a maximum and then decreases again as the specimen is rotated. If the refractive index of the mountant corresponds to the lower of the two refractive indices of the specimen then, as the specimen is rotated, it will become almost invisible, rapidly becoming more contrasty as its orientation changes, reaching a maximum at 90° to the original orientation. Further rotation will then cause the contrast to diminish again to a minimum at 180° and increase again to a maximum at 270° of rotation from the start.

An optically anisotropic (birefringent) uniaxial material may show the property called 'dichroism'. This means that the brightness and/or colour of the object will differ according to variation in the parts of the spectrum which are selectively absorbed from the light which it transmits; this in turn is related to the different permitted vibration directions of light in the material.

If a dichroic object is viewed with natural, unpolarized white light, no change will be seen when the object is rotated, since the light beams suffer the same absorption in each of the permitted vibration directions. If plane-polarized light is used to illuminate the specimen however, this light will be split into two components whose amplitudes will vary according to the permitted vibration directions of the polarizer and those of the specimen. This is shown in *Figure 5.1a*. Here, a plane-polarized beam of light (OP) enters a dichroic crystal with permitted vibration directions OA and OB. The amplitudes of the resultant emergent beams (OA' and OB') respectively, are given by dropping perpendiculars in turn from OP on to OA and OB. In this instance, as the angles POA and POB are both 45°, the two components OA' and OB' are equal. If we suppose that absorption due to the inherent properties of the material in the direction OA results in a dark brown colour and that in direction OB a light yellow colour, then in the situation illustrated, the material would appear in a colour intermediate between these two colours. If we now rotate the specimen clockwise through 30° (see *Figure 5.1b*), then amplitude OA' is much greater than OB'; since OA' is associated with the colour brown, this colour will predominate in the specimen. When the permitted vibration directions of the specimen are parallel with or perpendicular to those of the polarizer, then the only component which passes through the specimen is that parallel to the direction of the polarizer, with the result that one of the extreme absorption colours will be seen. Turning the specimen through 90° will allow the other colour to be seen.

Dichroism is most marked in some minerals such as crystals of tour-

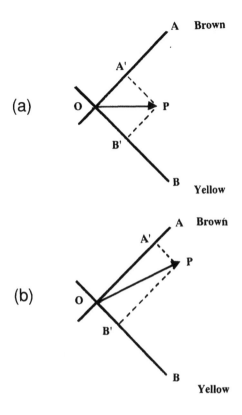

Figure 5.1: Effect of plane-polarized light.
   An illustration of the effect of illuminating a dichroic object with plane-polarized light vibrating in the direction OP. The object has two permitted vibration directions OA and OB. In diagram (a) the angles AOP and BOP are 45 degrees and the amplitudes of the resultant emergent beams OA' and OB' are equal. As absorption in direction OA gives a brown colour and that in OB a yellow, the resultant colour is intermediate between these. Rotation of the specimen by 30 degrees, as in (b), ensures that the resultant OB' is much less than OA' and the colour brown now predominates.

maline and biotite. The former is prismatic and uniaxial with the optic axis lying along the length of the crystal. This is parallel to the extraordinary vibration direction. Such crystals are blue, green or brown and appear darkest when their optic axis is at right angles to the plane of the polarizer; they are palest, therefore, when the long axis of the crystal lies parallel to the plane of vibration of the polarizer.

5.3 Observations between crossed polars; first-order red plate

As outlined in Section 5.1 above, if the polarizer and analyser are orientated at right angles to one another (i.e. 'crossed'), then the field of view of the microscope will appear dark unless a birefringent object is introduced in the correct orientation. In this case the polarized light will be resolved into two components which are polarized in mutually perpendicular planes. Since neither of these is at 90° to the analyser, some light will pass, and the object will appear light on a dark background. As the specimen is rotated with respect to the plane of polarization of the light, its brightness will change from maximally bright to completely dark. The polarizer provides light vibrating in an E–W direction, which passes through the specimen where it is split into two components vibrating at 90° to one another. In the case where each resulting component is vibrating at 45° to the vibration direction of the polarizer (i.e. NE–SW and SE–NW), the two components will have equal amplitudes, but will propagate with different velocities through the material, and so get progressively out of step by an amount which increases with the thickness of the crystal and the difference in the velocities. This 'out-of-stepness' can be expressed in various ways; the usual one is termed the optical path difference (OPD) which is equal to the thickness multiplied by the difference between the refractive indices, called the 'birefringence'. On emerging from the crystal the two components are said to 'recombine'. In reality, the rays are not suddenly 'split' and 'recombined', but optically the light behaves as if this were the case. This recombined light arrives at the analyser, which allows only light vibrating in the N–S direction to pass through. In considering this recombination we need to consider the OPD and the fact that white light consists of many wavelengths.

- For an OPD of zero, light which is vibrating in the E–W direction as it enters the object emerges from the object apparently unchanged; all of this light will then be blocked by the analyser (which is orientated to pass only light vibrating N–S).
- For OPDs which are small in relation to the wavelength of light, all colours of the spectrum pass through weakly, appearing as greyish-white light.
- As the OPD increases, the longer wavelengths of the spectral colours begin to dominate, and the colour changes through whitish-yellow, then orange, on to a distinctive deep purple-red or magenta called the 'sensitive tint'. These 'polarization colours', first studied by Newton (they are often known as Newton's colours), are not pure spectral colours but are mixtures of wavelengths. For example, the sensitive tint is white light with the middle (yellow-green) part of the spectrum removed.

- As the OPD increases still further the colours pass through a repeating sequence of 'orders'. Each successive order becomes less and less saturated, appearing much paler than those preceding it.

If the thickness of the specimen is known, the birefringence may be determined approximately by comparing the Newton's colour shown by the specimen with a chart of the colours (a Michel-Lévy chart). Conversely, if the birefringence is known then the thickness may be estimated.

Addition and subtraction of OPDs, or retardations, may be accomplished by superimposing two pieces of doubly refracting material. If these are arranged so that they appear bright between crossed polars, and their slower components (i.e. those that 'lag behind' the faster components) are both vibrating in the same direction, then the OPDs or retardations will add together. The resultant polarization colour will be higher (i.e. it will go *up* Newton's scale), representing the sum of that due to each component alone (see *Figure 5.2a*). If the materials are superimposed with their vibration directions at right angles (see *Figure 5.2b*), then the OPDs or retardations subtract and the colour will go *down* Newton's scale. Polarized-light microscopes are provided with accessories called compensators or 'retardation plates' to effect this change. A full explanation of these and their uses will be found in Hallimond (1970) or Robinson and Bradbury (1992).

For the accentuation of contrast, as opposed to quantitative determinations, only one such plate (called a 'selenite' or 'first-order red' plate) is normally used. This device is a thin slice of quartz, selenite or other birefringent material designed to introduce an OPD of exactly one wavelength when used with green light of 550 nm. When such a plate is placed at 45° between crossed polars, with no specimen in the field, light with a wavelength of 550 nm is extinguished so that the resultant colour is a brilliant purple-red or magenta. Because a tiny increase in retardation will alter the colour provided with the first-order red plate to blue, and an equally small decrease will change the colour to yellow, this compensator plate was formerly often called a 'sensitive tint' plate. For this reason the first-order red plate is used to detect very low order polarization colours, such as might occur with a weakly birefringent object placed between crossed polars. It will be remembered that if a birefringent specimen is orientated with its vibration directions parallel to either the polarizer or the analyser, the transmitted intensity of light will be zero. Hence in order to observe birefringence, the specimen must sit with its vibration directions at 45° to N–S and E–W. The retardation plate is made with its vibration directions along, and at right angles to, its long axis, therefore, for addition or subtraction to occur the plate must also be inserted at 45° to the N–S and E–W directions. When this is done, the specimen will appear either blue or yellow (according to whether there is addition or subtraction of the optical path difference) on a bright red field, and its anisotropy will thus be made very much more obvious. Thin sections of

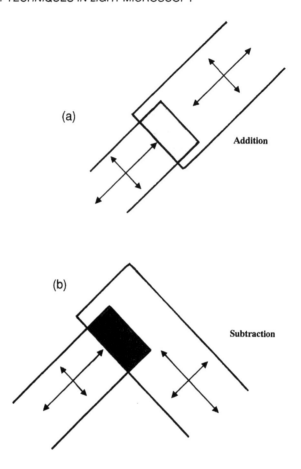

Figure 5.2: A diagram illustrating the effect of superimposing two doubly-refracting materials between crossed polars.

In (a) the fast directions of the material (indicated by the longer arrows) coincide, their retardations are added together, causing the perceived colour to go up Newton's scale (light tint). In (b) the reverse is true and the fast direction in one specimen is superimposed on the slow direction in the other. The retardations subtract; the effect is of an apparent thinning of the material and the colour goes down Newton's scale (as indicated by the darker tint).

minerals containing anisotropic crystals (for example calcite) may have a relatively high birefringence and be easy to see. Birefringent crystals are often found in certain plant cells, calcareous sponges, and some holo-thurians.

Most biological material, however, does not contain birefringent crystals but often shows a much weaker birefringence, due to the presence of orientated micelles contained in a matrix of different refractive index. Included in this category of 'form birefringence' would be that due to starch grains, many types of lipid droplets, some muscle fibres, collagen fibres and nerves. It is also possible for micelles of protein to become aligned when cytoplasmic streaming occurs and this 'flow birefringence' is often a marked feature of pseudopodia produced during amoeboid movement. In many biological objects showing form birefringence (such as living striated muscle fibres) the birefringence is low. In order to see such low degrees of birefringence, polars with high extinction factors are necessary. In such cases, use of the first-order red plate is a great advantage.

5.4 The use of polarized light in reflected-light microscopy

In reflected-light microscopy, the concepts which apply are similar to those outlined for transmitted light (see Section 5.3). The concept of refractive index (RI) is normally associated with light passing *through* an object, but it is also relevant to the *reflection* of light from the surface of an object. When light falls on a *non-absorbing* substance, part of the light is reflected but most of it is refracted. The amplitudes of the reflected and refracted components are determined by the RI, which applies not only to the light which is transmitted, but also to that which is reflected. In absorbing materials it is clearly the absorption which limits the amplitude of the transmitted beam, which only penetrates an extremely short distance into the specimen. Here again, the concepts of RI and absorption will describe not only the refracted beam (most of which is absorbed), but also the reflected beam which predominates and which concerns us here.

In a reflective anisotropic material, the plane-polarized light vibrating E–W is split into two components when it strikes the specimen. As before, when each component is vibrating at 45° to the vibration direction of the polarizer they will have equal amplitudes. These two components are reflected. The proportion of the incident light to that which is returned is called the reflectance (R), which is determined by the RI and the absorption of the material in each of these directions. The amplitude of the light reflected is determined by the values of the RI and the absorption of the specimen, both of which vary with direction. Furthermore, in opaque or absorbing materials the reflected components are out of step with each other, and this 'out-of stepness' can be expressed as an OPD in just the same way as with transmitted light. Newton's colours will be formed in the same way as already described for transmitted light. With reflecting materials, however, there is an added complication because dispersion varies according to wavelength (for many materials studied in transmission, dispersion is essentially constant), thus, dispersion provides a further source of colour in the image. This phenomenon is very important in practical microscopy of opaque minerals (ore microscopy); see Galopin and Henry (1972).

With incident light microscopy of some polished but unetched metal surfaces, such as zinc, beryllium or tin, the birefringence is again high and easy to see. In such circumstances polarized light may be of considerable help as a means of generating contrast and so showing up grain orientations very clearly. Some isotropic metals may be rendered anisotropic at their surfaces by adding an anodic oxide (in the case of aluminium) or sulphide film; alternatively special etching reagents may be used. Alpha brass etched in alcoholic ferric chloride is a good example of this, where anisotropy after deep etching is produced due to multiple oblique reflections formed in pits or furrows etched on to the surface of an isotropic crystal.

References

Bennett HS. (1950) The microscopical investigation of biological materials with polarized light. In *McClung's Handbook of Microscopical Technique* (ed. R McClung-Jones) (3rd edn). Hafner, New York, pp. 591–677.

Galopin R, Henry NFM. (1972) *Microscopic Study of Opaque Minerals.* Heffer, Cambridge.

Hallimond AF. (1970) *The Polarizing Microscope* (3rd edn). Vickers Instruments, York.

Mason CW. (1983) The study of double refractive materials by means of the polarizing microscope. In *Handbook of Chemical Microscopy* (ed. CW Mason) (4th edn) Vol. 1. John Wiley & Sons, New York, pp. 267–309.

Robinson PC, Bradbury S. (1992) *Qualitative Polarized Light Microscopy* (RMS Handbook no. 9). Oxford University Press, Oxford.

6 Phase Contrast and Modulation Contrast

Many important specimens, most particularly living unstained biological cells, are almost completely transparent. A typical preparation for study will consist of small membrane-bounded compartments containing aqueous fluid (the organelles), enclosed within a larger compartment of aqueous fluid of slightly different composition (the cell itself), the whole mounted either in fresh water, seawater, or an appropriate medium capable of supporting the life of cultured cells. The differences in light absorption between the various components of this preparation are negligible, and they will thus be quite invisible to the eye in bright-field transmitted-light microscopy. It is common practice in these circumstances to close down the illuminating aperture and defocus a little, as discussed in Section 3.1; there is a resulting increase in contrast (which can be considered to be a form of phase contrast) but the resolving power of the system will be seriously reduced. Although such specimens appear invisible in normal bright-field microscopy, they have in fact caused some small changes in the phase relationships between the rays of light as they emerge from the specimen, and they are thus frequently known as 'phase specimens'. The amount of this phase change, to which our eyes are not sensitive, is dependent upon the product of the refractive index of the object and its thickness. Only if such phase changes can be converted into amplitude changes will our eyes be able to appreciate the morphology of the object and contrast be generated.

The theory and practice of phase contrast were devised and developed by Frits Zernike (1934), for the testing of telescope mirrors; it was not until 1941 that the method was made available commercially for microscopy by Köhler and Loos working at the Zeiss laboratories. A paper on the application of phase contrast to the microscope was subsequently published by Zernike (1942a, b). After the Second World War microscopes incorporating phase contrast were marketed, and phase contrast rapidly became a major contrast technique.

Phase contrast provides an efficient method of enhancing the contrast of such specimens without unacceptable loss in resolution, and has proved itself extremely valuable in the study of dynamic events in living cells. The technique can also be applied to reflected light (Haynes, 1984), but this use has been largely superseded by newer methods of interference contrast.

Modulation contrast, another technique which enhances the contrast of phase specimens, is discussed in Section 6.6.

6.1 Theory of phase contrast

According to Abbe's theory, all specimens diffract light, and the information about their structure is carried by the diffracted beams. The direct, undiffracted light passes through the specimen without deviation, and reaches the image plane as a broad, expanding beam. The diffracted light also arrives in the primary image plane where an image of the object is formed. In the case of an absorbing specimen, the diffracted light which has passed through the specimen is half a wavelength (180°) out of phase with the direct light (the light which has passed through the background, or the specimen, without deviation due to diffraction); it is the interference between the diffracted and the direct beams which gives rise to the primary image (see *Figure 2.1*; the resultant beam in *Figure 6.1*). The imaging of non-absorbing, so-called 'phase' specimens such as a preparation of living cells, also takes place according to Abbe's theory but with one important difference. Since no contrast is seen in this image, we must conclude that there cannot be a half-wavelength phase difference between the diffracted and the direct beams making up the primary image. In fact, the diffracted beams, scattered at the interfaces between regions of rather small difference in refractive index, differ from the direct beams by about

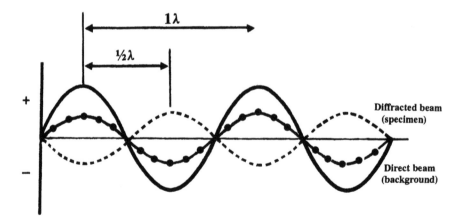

Figure 6.1: Amplitude objects.
  A diagram showing the direct beam passing through an amplitude object. The diffracted beam (originating at the specimen) is shown by a dashed line and is half a wavelength out of phase with the direct beam. The resultant beam (shown as a continuous line with superimposed black dots) is the sum of the direct (background) beam and the diffracted (specimen) beam. Note that this resultant is in phase with the direct beam but of lower amplitude.

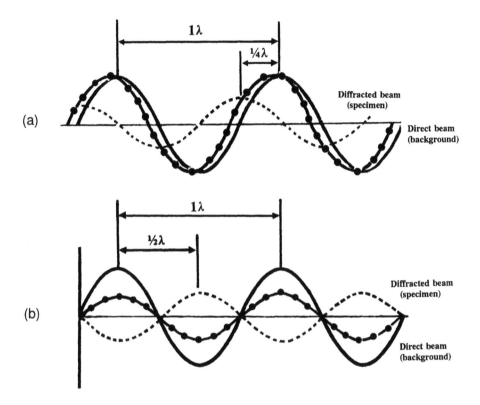

Figure 6.2: Phase objects.

(a) The direct, diffracted and resultant beams for a transparent, phase object. When the direct beam passes through a thin, transparent object, the resultant beam will show a small phase retardation with respect to that part of the direct beam which does not encounter the object. As with a transmitting object (see *Figure 6.1*), the resultant beam is derived from the sum of the direct (background) beam and the diffracted (specimen) beam. This diffracted beam is shown as a dashed line in the diagram and it can be seen that it is one quarter of a wavelength out of phase with the direct beam. (b) If a further one quarter wavelength retardation is added in the microscope to the diffracted beam, so shifting the curve for that beam (shown by the dashed line) a further quarter of a wavelength to the left, a total retardation of one half-wavelength with respect to the direct beam gives the situation illustrated. Discerning readers will observe that these curves are identical to those shown in *Figure 6.1* for an amplitude object. In fact, the image of the transparent *phase object* has been transformed into a *simulated amplitude object* with sufficient contrast for it to be clearly seen.

one quarter of a wavelength, a difference which cannot result in amplitude contrast due to interference (see *Figure 6.2a*). An explanation of the origin of this quarter-wavelength phase difference may be beyond the needs of the reader, and is not essential to the understanding of the technique; those who wish to consider phase contrast more deeply should read the short account in the Appendix which outlines an approach using vectors (considered more fully in the papers by Barer, listed in the references.

The paper of 1959 is perhaps more accessible to those readers who are less mathematically inclined).

In the phase-contrast technique as devised by Zernike, the phase difference between the direct and the diffracted rays, and their relative amplitudes, can be altered to produce the most favourable conditions for interference and to increase contrast. Essentially, his system causes the beams diffracted by the specimen to pass through a slightly longer optical path than the direct light; this optical path difference is arranged to be one quarter of a wavelength. Thus, when the diffracted beams come together with the direct light to form the primary image there is half a wavelength phase difference between them: one quarter-wavelength due to diffraction by the specimen and another quarter-wavelength resulting from the technique (see *Figure 6.2b*). This provides a situation similar to that of the absorbing specimen, where a half-wavelength phase difference gives rise to considerable contrast when the beams interfere to form the primary image; we have thus contrived to make our transparent phase specimen behave as if it were an amplitude (absorbing) specimen.

6.2   The construction of the phase-contrast microscope

Over the 50 years during which phase-contrast microscopy has been commercially available, the theoretical requirements have been realized in several ways. All manufacturers now agree on the basic method about to be described; some other, older methods will be discussed in the next section.

In a Köhler illumination system the source of light, usually the lamp filament, is imaged into the lower focal plane of the condenser, where the illuminating aperture diaphragm is normally fitted. In a phase-contrast system an annular diaphragm is placed here to provide a hollow cone of light with its apex at the specimen, which enters the objective as an inverted hollow cone (see *Figure 6.3*). An image of the illuminating annulus appears in the next conjugate plane, the back focal plane of the objective, in the form of a ring of light.

The next essential requirement for a phase-contrast system is the inclusion of a device, generally called a phase plate, capable of selectively altering the phase of the direct, undiffracted light with respect to the diffracted light. This phase plate is usually fitted within the objective, in its back focal plane, where the image of the illuminating annulus falls upon it. In the area covered by the image of the illuminating annulus, the phase plate is arranged to have an optical path which is usually one quarter of a wavelength shorter than that through the remainder of its area; we shall call this optically modified area of the phase plate the *phase ring*. The phase ring is represented in the diagram (*Figure 6.4*) as an annular trench or flat-topped ridge, although it may take other forms in modern manufacture. In the absence of a diffracting specimen, all the light from the condenser will pass through the phase ring; a diffracting specimen, on the other hand, will deviate some of the light from this path, causing it to pass through the optically thicker part of the phase plate. In this case, the phase plate thus adds a second quarter-wavelength phase difference selectively to the diffracted light, resulting in a half-wavelength difference when the direct and diffracted light combine in the primary image plane. If the pattern of light diffracted from a typical phase specimen is examined, it will be seen that the direct beam is considerably brighter than the diffracted beams. The brightness of the direct beam must be reduced to

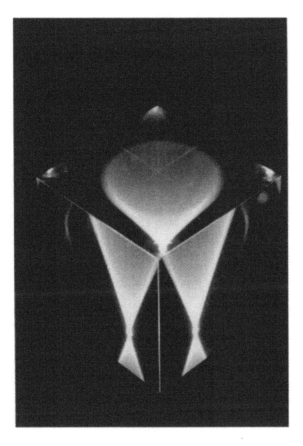

Figure 6.3: Light path produced by a phase-contrast condenser.

A photograph of a turbid glass cube to show the inverted hollow cone of light which arises from the annular diaphragm in a phase-contrast condenser. The camera was directed towards one corner of the cube in order to show a side view of the hollow cone through two vertical faces and a section of the cone of light appearing on the top surface.

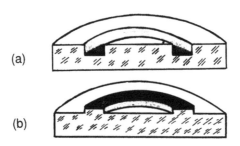

Figure 6.4: Diagrams of phase plates.

Diagrams of phase plates in section to show the phase ring with its absorbing layer in the form of an annular groove (a) for positive phase contrast, or annular ridge (b) for negative phase contrast. This would be included either on a plate in the back focal plane of the objective or applied to one of the lens elements lying close to that plane.

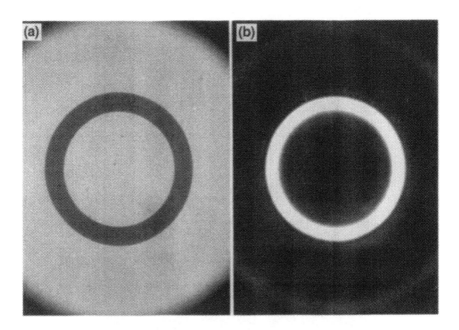

Figure 6.5: Photographs of phase plates *in situ*.

(a) A photograph of the phase plate *in situ* in an objective, showing the phase ring by virtue of its absorbing layer. (b) A photograph of the same objective as in *Figure 6.5a*, now illuminated with the ring of light deriving from a matching phase-contrast condenser.

make it similar to that of the diffracted beams, to enable the diffracted light, once its phase has been changed, to interfere and provide maximum contrast in the image. The phase ring (that area of the phase plate which is conjugated with the illuminating annulus) is thus not only made with a different optical path from its surroundings, but also with a different transmission to reduce the amplitude of the direct or zero-order beam. Usually this is achieved by the evaporative deposition of an extremely thin layer of an absorbing substance. It is of course this difference in transmission, rather than its difference in optical path, that enables the phase ring to be seen when looking into the rear of the objective (see *Figure 6.5*).

Because a range of different objectives will have different focal lengths (magnifications) and apertures, a phase-contrast condenser usually has several illuminating annuli mounted interchangeably on a rotating turntable. An empty space is also provided, often fitted with an iris diaphragm, to enable the condenser to be used for normal bright-field microscopy. A phase-contrast condenser may also carry devices for dark ground and differential interference contrast (DIC; see Chapter 7).

It is obviously necessary that the image of the illuminating annulus should be precisely coincident with the phase ring in the objective. Phase-contrast objectives must be used with a condenser designed for them, so that the annulus image will be of the correct size, and adjustment for concentricity must also be provided. This generally takes the form of two centring screws or other devices, set at 90° or 120° to one another, by which the annulus may be moved to coincide with the axis of the phase ring. In order to observe the progress of this adjustment, it is necessary to examine the back focal plane of the objective. The simplest method for this is the use of a device variously known as a 'phase telescope', 'auxiliary telescope' or 'auxiliary microscope'. The telescope consists of a two lenses, arranged to act as the objective and eyepiece of an optical system intermediate between a telescope and a microscope, hence the confusion about the terminology. This 'telescope' is focused on about 150 mm so that when it is inserted into the microscope tube in place of the eyepiece, it provides a magnified view of the back focal plane of the objective. A more sophisticated device to achieve a similar aim is the Bertrand lens, built into microscopes intended primarily for use with polarized light, which can be inserted between the objective lens and the eyepiece. The Bertrand lens acts as a relay lens, transferring an image of the back focal plane of the objective into the plane within the eyepiece normally occupied by the primary image; this enables the back focal plane to be observed through the normal eyepiece(s). Both telescope and Bertrand lens must be fitted with a focusing adjustment, since the back focal planes of objectives of different magnifications (different focal lengths) lie at different levels within the microscope. Using a well-designed system, the centration adjustment should be substantially correct for all objectives in a matched set, and should remain unchanged unless the adjustments of the microscope are disturbed.

The phase-contrast technique relies on the phase ring adding a quarter-wavelength phase difference between direct and diffracted beams. Microscopes are, however, generally used with light of wavelengths ranging from approximately 450 nm up to 750 nm, where one quarter of the larger value is not far from one half of the smaller one. Phase-contrast objectives are specified to operate optimally at one particular wavelength, commonly 550 nm. Light of this wavelength appears green, the colour to which our eyes are most sensitive and for which lens aberrations have been best corrected. A set of equipment for phase contrast will normally include a filter of the appropriate colour. Objectives built to operate with other wavelengths, in the ultra-violet range for example, have been made, although these would need to be specially ordered from the manufacturer. It must be remarked, however, that the phase-shift occurring at the specimen is only precisely one quarter of a wavelength for a specimen with virtually no optical path difference from its surroundings. In practice for most specimens, therefore, the use of one precise waveband should not be regarded as obligatory except in extreme circumstances; satisfactory results can usually be obtained using white light, photographed using colour film if desired.

6.3 Variants of phase contrast

The most commonly used system described above, where the diffracted rays traverse an optical path one-quarter wavelength longer than that of the direct rays, is known as 'positive' phase contrast. Features having refractive indices higher than those of their surroundings will give rise to diffracted beams one-quarter of a wavelength retarded with respect to the direct beam; a further one quarter wavelength retardation at the phase plate, giving a total of one half a wavelength retardation, will cause these more-highly refracting features to appear darker in the image. This explains the appearance of the image of a living cell (see *Figure 6.6*), where the nucleus and other structures all have higher refractive indices and appear darker than their surroundings (see also *Figure 6.8*).

Phase plates can also be built in which the phase ring has the longer optical path, so that the diffracted rays are advanced in phase with respect to the direct beam. They now interfere constructively, causing more highly refractile features to appear bright against a darker background. Because this is the inverse of the common situation, the system is known as negative phase contrast. The degree of absorption of the phase ring (generally approximately 75%) is another variable. Anoptral contrast, formerly produced by Reichert, is a form of negative phase contrast in which the absorbance of the phase ring is high, about 90%; this system provided an image showing more refractile features as bright against a relatively dark, brownish background.

It is not necessary for the phase-changing area of the phase plate to be in the form of a ring, although for reasons of azimuthal symmetry a ring is the obvious pattern; in the early days of the phase-contrast technique, the firm of C. Baker produced a design with a cross-shaped phase-changing

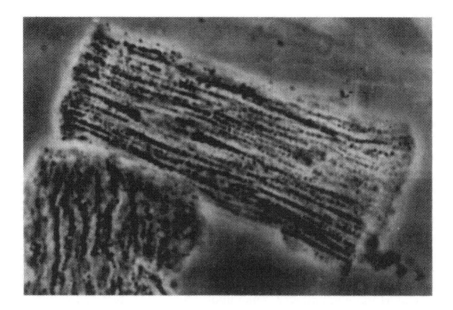

Figure 6.6: Phase-contrast photograph of cardiac myocytes.
A photograph by positive phase contrast of isolated cardiac myocytes mounted in saline. Note the ample contrast, and that the cells and their inclusions are surrounded by the characteristic bright 'halo'.

area. This simplified the mechanical design of the condenser, since just one cross in the condenser could serve the needs of several objectives with a range of magnifications and apertures; unfortunately, this system produced a serious image artefact, since out-of-focus features all appeared as disturbing, small crosses.

In another variant, still manufactured today and intended particularly for inverted microscopes, the phase plates are not built into the back focal plane of the objectives. An image of the back focal plane is relayed by an extra lens system into a position just beneath the binocular head, where phase plates may be inserted on a suitable slider. This system has the advantage of providing phase-contrast imaging without requiring the purchase of a second and special set of objectives.

Condensers operating according to a different principle were manufactured by Leitz (the Heine condenser) and Reichert (the Polyphos) amongst others. These condensers, which included reflecting as well as refracting components in their design, produced a hollow cone of light of variable included angle, such that they could be adjusted to suit phase-contrast objectives across the whole range. In addition to phase contrast, with only a minor adjustment, they could provide bright field with the cone of light falling within the objective aperture but not upon the phase ring, and also dark ground with the cone of light adjusted to be more oblique than the objective aperture.

6.4 The phase-contrast image

A microscope image frequently does not resemble its object. Phase-contrast images clearly fall into this category: the objects are invisible, and the aim of the technique is to produce visible images of them. The simple act of increasing contrast does not in itself produce an obviously disturbing artefact leading to misinterpretation: a similar effect might result from suitable staining, for example. However, phase contrast images suffer from other artefacts which can prove troublesome, particularly where features are measured using an automatic system for image analysis.

The phase-contrast image is formed by interference between light which has undergone a phase change as a result of passing through features in the object, and the light which has passed through unaffected. The separation between these two categories of light, enabling their relative phase to be changed, relies on diffraction by the fine details of the object, which causes light that has encountered the object to pass outside the phase ring. Unfortunately, however, some light which has interacted with the coarser features of the object will be diffracted through an angle too small to cause it to pass outside the phase ring (which in the ideal but impractical case would be of infinitely small width), and light will be diffracted by some finer features to fall on another part of the phase ring. These effects, together with a complex of other factors, lead to the formation of the halo around objects which appear bright (and vice versa), which is characteristic of phase-contrast images. In the positive phase-contrast image in *Figure 6.6*, the cell (an isolated cardiac myocyte) and the more highly-refractile internal features (mitochondria) are all surrounded by a bright halo and lined with a dark halo; negative phase contrast produces the opposite effects. One result of this is that the positions of the edges of these features cannot be determined precisely.

In addition to the halo, phase contrast suffers from other limitations which can lead to difficulties in interpretation. The contrast effect is maximal at regions of sharp change in optical path ('edges'), and relatively low where there are slow changes ('wedges'). The contrast effect thus reduces towards the centre of objects which present a uniform optical path, an effect sometimes known as 'shading off', and thus the centre of one region will appear the same shade of grey as the centre of another region of different refractive index.

A further characteristic of the phase contrast image is that thick specimens show reduced contrast, which periodically reverses with increasing thickness. This is because light passing through thicker specimens either achieves a phase difference of more than the typical one quarter of a wavelength, or suffers multiple interactions with several features. Hence, the ideal specimen for phase contrast is extremely thin, or at least highly transparent. As a consequence of these effects, the interpretation of phase-contrast images is not straightforward, especially when unaccompanied by information from other techniques.

Since the phase-contrast image is a result of the difference between the refractive index (RI) of the object and that of its surroundings, no contrast will be seen when these indices are identical, and an object that appears dark when surrounded by a medium of *lower* RI will appear bright within a medium of higher RI. Contrast in the phase-contrast image is thus very sensitive to the relationship between the object and its mounting medium, a factor which is now inadequately understood or exploited by microscopists. Many living cells can, without detriment, be mounted in media whose RI can be adjusted by varying concentrations of a suitable protein (e.g. saline with bovine serum albumen added), resulting in useful variations in contrast. The effect on image contrast of differences of RI forms the basis of the technique of immersion refractometry (Barer and Ross, 1952), by which the RI of cell cytoplasm can be determined by comparison with a range of media of known RI (again mixtures of saline and bovine serum albumen). Since most of the important organic substances found within living cells have similar specific refractive index increments, RI measurements by this method provide useful information on the concentrations of intracellular substances.

6.5 Phase contrast in reflected light

Both phase contrast and modulation contrast (see Section 6.6) can, in principle, be applied to reflected-light microscopy, although neither technique is currently in common use. Both techniques are achieved in bright-field epi-illumination in a manner comparable to their transmitted-light counterparts, modified to take account of the fact that the objective lens acts also as the condenser.

For phase contrast, the illuminating annulus obviously cannot be situated within the objective lens, since it would obstruct the imaging rays; to avoid this, an *image* of the annulus is projected into the back focal plane of the objective, where the phase plate would normally be located. In practice, there is also another difference from the typical transmitted-light system: the phase plate is not fitted in the back focal plane of the objective, but in an *image* of the back focal plane formed by the inclusion of an additional lens system. This provides several important advantages:

- It avoids disturbing reflections and scattered light which would be caused by passing the relatively bright ring of illumination through the phase ring.
- It provides greater brightness because the illuminating rays do not pass

through the absorbing region of the phase plate while on their way to the specimen.

- It enables one set of objective lenses to be used optimally for phase-contrast and bright-field applications.
- It makes it possible for one common phase plate to be used for all objectives.

This last feature requires the lens system which forms the image of the back focal plane to be an adjustable one, so that objectives of a range of apertures can be accommodated with one common phase plate.

Whereas in transmission the diffracted light acquires its phase shift at the edges of features in the object because of the different refractive indices of these features, this cannot occur with opaque specimens. In reflected-light phase contrast, these phase-differences are caused by relief on the specimen surface: features which are higher than their surroundings appear darker in positive phase contrast, and vice versa.

6.6 Modulation contrast

Modulation contrast, devised by Hoffman and Gross (1975a, b, 1977), is a technique of contrast enhancement which is relatively simple to install on a conventional microscope. Like phase contrast, it enhances the contrast of unstained, phase specimens, but it is sensitive to *gradients* of optical path length, rather than to sudden discontinuities of refractive index. Unlike phase contrast, it produces an asymmetrical, directional image; phase gradients in one direction are always rendered bright, and those in the opposite direction dark. This gives a pseudo-three-dimensional effect which must not be misinterpreted as relief in the object, since it represents variations in optical density rather than topography. In this respect the modulation-contrast image is similar to that from differential interference contrast, but the optical principles are completely different.

6.7 Construction of the modulation-contrast microscope

A device known as a modulator plate is fitted in the back focal plane of the objective. In the original form, shown in *Figure 6.7a*, this consists of a glass plate with areas of three degrees of transmittance: approximately one third is fully transmitting; there is then a central stripe of grey (15%

transmission) with the remaining third as a dark grey (1% transmission) area. Using a construction similar to that for phase contrast, the condenser is fitted with a slit in its lower focal plane, positioned so that its image falls on the grey area of the modulator plate. Light undeviated by the specimen will thus pass through the grey area of the modulator, where its intensity will be reduced to about 15% of the original. If phase gradients are considered to be a series of tiny prisms, it will be seen that a slope in one direction will refract light away from the slit into the clear part of the modulator plate giving rise to a bright area in the image, while a slope in the opposite direction will divert light into the dark apart of the modulator. Because the illumination is strongly azimuthal, as it is produced by a slit positioned away from the optical axis, the system is strongly directional and the appearance of an image will depend upon the orientation of the slit relative to the phase gradients of the object. It will frequently be helpful to rotate the object (ideally with a rotating stage), in order to observe the separate effects due to the directionality of the imaging system and the structure of the specimen. The resolution of modulation contrast is equivalent to that of a standard objective used with full-cone illumination.

In a later paper (Hoffman, 1977) the system is modified from the original in that much more of the modulator is left clear (i.e. with 100% transmission) and it has narrower dark and grey regions (see *Figure 6.7b*). The slit in the diaphragm fitted in the condenser front focal plane is also reduced in length and is half covered by a strip of polarizing material (see *Figure 6.7c*). If a polarizer is fitted below the diaphragm, rotation of the polarizer with respect to the slit will vary the effective slit width. When the polars are crossed, the slit will be appear narrow and can be imaged entirely on the grey area of the modulator (G in *Figure 6.7b*); the resultant modulation-contrast image will show very high contrast and a high degree of coherence. The use of the narrow slit gives good images of thin, flat objects in which the differences in phase gradient are small. If the polar is orientated with its vibration direction parallel to that in the slit, then the effective slit width is much greater and its image on the modulator plate will fall not only on the grey portion but also, in part, on the bright area (B in *Figure 6.7b*). This will reduce the image contrast and coherence and give much better images of thicker objects where large differences in RI exist, as in mounts of fresh human red blood cells. Modulation contrast provides:

- a 3-D appearance to the image
- optical sectioning
- directional sensitivity to optical gradients
- optimal imaging
- increased contrast and control of coherence

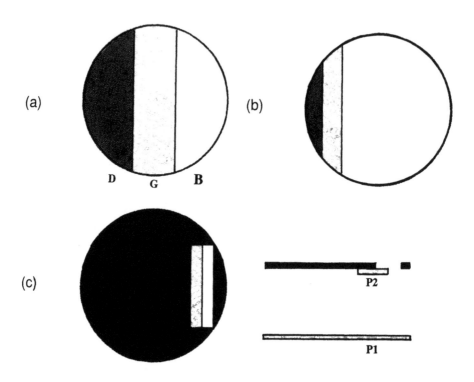

Figure 6.7: A diagram of the method for producing modulation contrast.
(a) The original form of the disc introduced into the back focal plane of the objective. The bright area (B) was clear, the grey area (G) had a transmittance of 15% and the dark area (D) transmitted only 1% of the light. This disc was used with a central slit diaphragm in the condenser front focal plane. An image of this slit was arranged to fall on the grey area G. (b) The later form of asymmetrical objective disc designed for use with a modified condenser diaphragm and a polarizer in the substage. (c) The condenser diaphragm designed for use with the modulator shown in (b) above. It has an offset slit partially covered by 'Polaroid' (P2). This diaphragm is used with a separate polarizer preceding it in the illumination path to allow an effective variation in the width of the slit. When the polarizers are crossed, the effective illuminating slit is narrow and its image falls within the grey area of the modulator disc. If the polarizers are parallel, the slit is effectively wider and is imaged also on to part of the bright area of the modulator; this allows the user to vary the image contrast.

The very limited depth of field provided by this technique allows effective optical sectioning of objects preventing details above and below the plane of focus from obscuring or blurring the image. This is well illustrated in the paper already cited (Hoffman, 1977), where photographs of human buccal epithelial cell are shown. Unlike phase-contrast images, those produced by modulation contrast do not have a halo; the appearance of the two types of image is very different and each provides different information. The phase-contrast system converts optical path differences to amplitude variations in the image plane, whilst modulation contrast converts phase gradients to amplitude differences – these two microscope systems complement rather than compete with each other.

Zeiss have recently introduced a new contrast technique which appears to have some characteristics in common with modulation contrast; this is called VAREL or variable relief contrast. Special objectives combine a phase plate with a conventional phase ring for phase contrast with a peripheral band of absorbing material for the VAREL technique. The first focal plane of the condenser carries a slider bearing both a standard phase-contrast illuminating annulus and a special diaphragm for VAREL. This contains two crescent shaped apertures, one on the left and one on the right, which can be displaced laterally by a variable amount so that the image of one of them falls on the absorbing region of the VAREL ring in the objective back focal plane. In this way the relief contrast giving an illusion of the third dimension may be adjusted to make the specimen appear to be illuminated from one side or the other. The technique provides a relatively inexpensive and effective alternative to phase contrast, modulation contrast or differential interference contrast. It is currently fitted to inverted microscopes intended for the examination of cells in culture on microtitre plates.

6.8   Setting-up phase contrast

A microscope with one or more phase-contrast objectives is required, in addition to the following pieces of equipment:

- A special phase-contrast condenser, or one into which a suitable annulus may be fitted.
- An 'auxiliary microscope' or 'telescope', usually provided with the phase-contrast kit (not required where the microscope is fitted with a Bertrand lens).
- A green filter (optional).

1. Set up the microscope for Köhler illumination in bright-field using the lowest magnification phase-contrast objective and a stained specimen, ensuring that the condenser is centred using the normal condenser centring screws.
2. Exchange the specimen for an unstained, phase specimen.
3. Remove an eyepiece, replace it with the 'telescope', and use the latter's adjustment to focus on the phase ring in the back focal plane of the objective, (where a Bertrand lens is fitted, this should be inserted and focused, with no need to disturb the eyepiece).
4. Move the appropriate illuminating annulus into position in the condenser. The positions on the turntable of annuli in the condenser are usually marked with the objective's magnification or with a reference number (e.g. Ph2 in the Zeiss system).

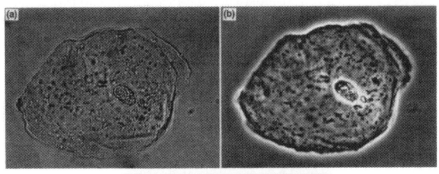

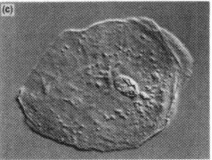

Figure 6.8: An epithelial cell imaged in three modes.
The same unstained buccal epithelial cell (which measures approximately 150 µm across) imaged in three different modes. (a) By means of restricted direct light resulting from closure of the illuminating aperture diaphragm. Contrast has been obtained at the expense of resolution. (b) By positive phase contrast; note the strong 'halo' around the periphery of both the cell and the nucleus. (c) By means of differential interference contrast (see Chapter 7). Although the appearance suggests the third dimension, this is an optical artefact of the technique.

5. While observing through the telescope (or Bertrand lens), centre the image of the annulus precisely on the phase ring using the adjusting devices provided. These will be a pair of screws or levers; do not disturb the normal condenser centring adjustments.
6. Remove the telescope, replace the eyepiece (remove the Bertrand lens) and focus the image using the fine adjustment.
7. Insert the green filter if desired.
8. On changing to another objective, it will usually be necessary to change to the appropriate illuminating annulus also. Repeat steps 3, 5 and 6 as necessary.

6.9   Setting-up modulation contrast

A microscope with one or more modulation contrast objectives is required, in addition to the following pieces of equipment:

- A special modulation-contrast condenser, or one into which a suitable slit diaphragm may be fitted.
- A polarizer if the illuminating slit has a polarizing area incorporated.
- An 'auxiliary microscope' or 'telescope' (not required where the microscope is fitted with a Bertrand lens).

1. With the slit diaphragm and polarizer (if used) removed, set up the microscope for Köhler illumination in bright field using the lowest magnification modulation-contrast objective and a stained specimen, ensuring that the condenser is centred using the normal condenser centring screws.
2. Exchange the specimen for an unstained specimen.
3. Remove an eyepiece, replace it with the 'telescope', and use the telescope's focusing adjustment to focus on the modulator plate in the back focal plane of the objective (where a Bertrand lens is fitted, this should be inserted and focused, with no need to disturb the eyepiece).
4. Move the appropriate slit diaphragm into position in the condenser. While observing through the telescope (or Bertrand lens), adjust the illuminating slit so that its image falls on to the grey region of the modulator plate using the adjusting devices provided. These may be a pair of screws or levers; do not disturb the normal condenser centring adjustments. If the modulator plate has a polarizing region, insert the polarizer and rotate until the narrowest image of the illuminating slit is obtained. Remove the telescope and replace the eyepiece (remove the Bertrand lens) and focus the image using the fine adjustment. Rotate the polarizer to adjust contrast as desired.
5. On changing to another objective, it will usually be necessary to change the illuminating diaphragm and repeat steps 3, 4, 5, 7 and 8 as necessary.

References

Barer R. (1952a) A vector theory of phase contrast and interference contrast. I Positive phase contrast. *J. R. Microsc. Soc.* **72**, 10–38.

Barer R. (1952b) A vector theory of phase contrast and interference contrast. II Positive phase contrast (continued). *J. R. Microsc. Soc.* **72**, 81–88.

Barer R. (1953a) A vector theory of phase contrast and interference microscopy. III Negative phase contrast. *J. R. Microsc. Soc.* **73**, 30–39.

Barer R. (1953b) A vector theory of phase contrast and intererence contrast. IV Type B phase contrast. *J. R. Microsc. Soc.* **73**, 206–215.

Barer R. (1959) Phase, interference and polarizing microscopy. In *Analytical Cytology* (ed. RC Mellors) (2nd edn). McGraw Hill, New York, pp. 169–272.

Barer R, Ross KFA. (1952) The refractometry of living cells. *J. Physiol.* **118**, 38.

Haynes R. (1984) *Optical Microscopy of Materials.* International Textbook Co., London.

Hoffman R, Gross L. (1975a) The modulation contrast microscope. *Nature* **254**, 586–588.

Hoffman R, Gross L. (1975b) Modulation contrast microscope. *Appl. Optics* **14**, 1169–1176.

Hoffman R. (1977) The modulation contrast microscope: principles and performance. *J. Microsc.* **110**, 205–222.

Zernike F. (1934) Diffraction theory of the knife-edge test and its improved form, the phase-contrast method. *R. Astron. Soc. Monthly Notices* **94**, 377–384.

Zernike F. (1942a) Phase-contrast, a new method for the microscopic observation of transparent objects. Part I. *Physica* **9**, 686–698.

Zernike F. (1942b) Phase-contrast, a new method for the microscopic observation of transparent objects. Part II. *Physica* **9**, 974–986.

7 Interference Contrast

Phase-contrast microscopy has for many years been the preferred method for enhancing contrast due to differences in refractive index between the object and its mounting medium. However, the phase differences between the light diffracted by the object and that which is unaffected may also be converted into amplitude differences by the use of some form of interference microscope. Interference is, of course, an important factor in the formation of all microscope images: in bright field and phase contrast, interference occurs amongst the beams diffracted by the object, and also between these beams and the light that passes through the specimen without deviation. In these cases the beams which interfere, as well as acquiring their differences in phase from their interactions with the object, have also been separated by the object and thus caused to take their different paths through the microscope. Instruments generally known as 'interference microscopes' are different in that the separation of light into beams which will interfere is actually carried out by the optical system of the microscope, before the light encounters the specimen. In these instruments, each illuminating ray is split into two beams which are coherent one with the other, and thus subsequently capable of interference when recombined.

The earlier interference microscopes, designed principally for measurement of optical path differences, are often known as interferometers. In these, one beam, known as the object beam because it has been modified by interaction with the object, is combined with another beam, the reference beam, which has followed a path in which it has not encountered the object. A class of instruments developed more recently, usually called differential interference microscopes, are used principally for contrast enhancement.

The most important difference between different designs of interference microscope is the way in which the reference beam is separated from the object beam. There are three fundamental possibilities, shown diagrammatically in *Figures 7.1* and *7.2*.

(a) The beams are separated so that only one of them meets the specimen (see *Figure 7.1a, b, c; Figure 7.2a*).
(b) Both beams meet the specimen but only one of them interacts with the object within it (see *Figure 7.2a*).
(c) Both beams interact with the object itself (see *Figure 7.2b, c*).

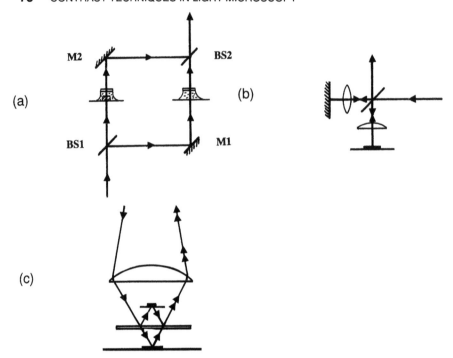

Figure 7.1:   Schematic diagrams of interference microscopes showing object and reference beams.

(a) Mach-Zehnder or 'round-the-square' system using simple semi-reflecting beam splitters to divide and recombine the beam. For further details see the text. (b) The principle of the Linnik interferometer for epi-illumination; the beam is divided by a semi-reflecting beam splitter and the reference beam is returned from a mirror. (c) The Mirau system in which the beam splitter/combiner and the reference surface are all carried on, or in, the objective lens.

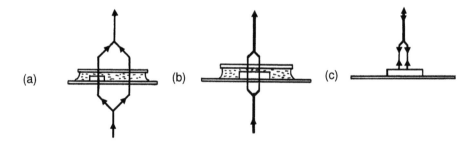

Figure 7.2:   Schematic diagrams of interference microscopes showing objects and reference beams.

(a) The Smith double image system in which the beam is divided before passing through the specimen into two beams, one of which acts as object beam whilst the other is the reference beam which by-passes the object. The beams are relatively widely separated and result in a double image of the object. (b) Differential interference contrast for transmitted light. The separation between the two beams is very small; consequently, although both interact with the object itself there is no doubling of the image. (c) Differential interference contrast for epi-illumination. Again, there is only a small separation between the beams and both interact with the object itself.

Here we are using the word *object* to refer to the item from which the microscope's image is formed, and *specimen* to refer to the preparation in general,that is the slide, mountant and coverglass.

Interference microscopes have been classified in more detail by Pluta (1993) as follows:

1. Only one beam carries an image of the object under study; the reference beam has no contact with the object. Systems of this type include the Linnik, Mach-Zehnder, Watson and Mirau (see *Figure 7.1a, b, c*).
2. Both beams carry an image of the object, but one of them is strongly out of focus, superimposed on the in-focus image, and acts as the reference beam. The Smith double-focus microscope belongs to this category.
3. Both beams carry an image of the object; the reference image is out of focus as in 2 above, but is laterally displaced. Two images of the object are formed. The Smith double-image shearing microscope is an example of this system (see *Figure 7.2a*).
4. Both beams carry a sharp image of the object, laterally displaced so that the clear background to the object in one image acts as the reference for the other, and vice versa.
5. Both beams carry a sharp image of the object, as in 4 above, but they are laterally displaced through a distance smaller than the minimum resolved distance of the objective (see *Figure 7.2b, c*). Differential interference contrast (DIC) microscopes, including those after Nomarski, belong to this category.

The principle of the interference microscope is perhaps easiest to understand by considering the Mach-Zehnder system, sometimes called a 'round the square' system and shown in diagrammatic form in *Figure 7.1a*. The light from a common source is split by means of a semi-reflecting plate (BS1) into two beams, one of which is reflected from a fully-reflecting mirror (M1) so that it is parallel to the original beam. The original beam is reflected by a second fully-reflecting mirror (M2) on to a second semi-reflecting beam-splitter (BS2) where it recombines with (and interferes with) the other beam. If one beam passes through the object mounted on the slide and the other only through a matching slide, mountant and coverslip, then any phase change introduced by the object will be represented as an interference pattern which can be visualized. A microscope system such as this naturally requires matched condenser/objective pairs and hence is cumbersome and expensive; Leitz formerly manufactured an instrument constructed on these principles. The final interference pattern could be adjusted for either a uniform or a fringed field.

    An alternative method of dividing and recombining a beam of light makes use of birefringent crystals and requires only a single microscope optical system; an interferometer using this principle was described over a century ago by Jamin and later applied to the microscope by Lebedeff.

Such systems allow control of the amplitude and phase relationships of the two beams, both of which pass through the slide on the stage, by means of polars and birefringent compensating plates inserted in the appropriate place in the optical path. The basic principle of such instruments is shown in *Figure 7.3*. The separation between the beams (x in the diagram) is relatively large and so a double image of each object is formed. Practical realization of this principle was achieved by Francis Smith (see *Figure 7.5*) using Wollaston prisms to act as beam splitter and combiner; many instruments designed by him and manufactured by Baker, Cooke Troughton & Simms, and Vickers are still extant. Microscopes of this type produce double images, in which the contrast is a function of the optical path differences between the object and its surroundings.

While eminently suitable for their prime purpose of measurement of optical path differences due to variations in mass and thickness (in transmission) or height (in reflected light), these systems produce images which are often not easily interpretable, and are not generally suitable for simple, qualitative enhancement of contrast; perhaps as a consequence most of them are rarely encountered except in specialist laboratories. The system of interference microscopy in greatest use today, and which in many cases has superseded phase contrast for qualitative enhancement of contrast, is differential interference contrast (DIC), in particular the system patented by Nomarski in 1953. The DIC image shows characteristic pronounced 'relief', or a shadowed effect, which results both from surface irregularities and from optical path differences in a transparent object. The use of DIC with high numerical aperture objectives also results in a very shallow depth of field so that out-of-focus details produce much less impairment of image sharpness than in many other techniques.

7.1 Differential interference contrast

The essential feature of DIC, in comparison to the instruments discussed above, is that *both* interfering beams pass through or reflect from the object, separated by an extremely small distance, which is arranged to be less than the minimum resolved distance of the objective. It is not apparent to the observer that the image is made up of these two superimposed components, since their separation is too small to be resolved. Each point in the image, however, is made up from two beams of light from closely adjacent parts of the object, and a phase difference will exist between the members of each pair of beams, depending on their respective optical paths due to their interaction with the object; the two beams are no longer separately identifiable as object and reference beams. The contrast is described as differential, using this word as in mathematics, since it is a function of the rate of change of optical path across the object; the steeper the gradient of optical path at the boundary of a feature, the greater the contrast,

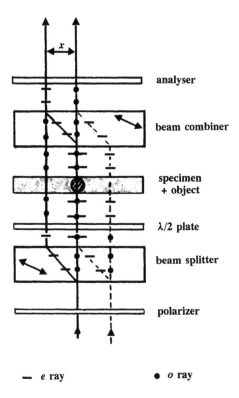

analyser

beam combiner

specimen
+ object

$\lambda/2$ plate

beam splitter

polarizer

— e ray   ● o ray

Figure 7.3: The Jamin-Lebedeff interference system.
    The object and reference beams are separated by means of birefringent plates operating on plane-polarized light. There is a relatively large separation (x) between the beams and this gives rise to a double image of the object.After passage through the specimen the beams are recombined by means of another birefringent plate and an analyser.

(it may be convenient to remember that contrast in DIC is due to 'wedges', whereas in phase contrast it is due to 'edges'). In the case of transmitting objects the optical path differences result from gradients of refractive index and/or thickness; in the case of reflected light, gradients of topography have the same effect. The construction and operation of the DIC microscope will be described first for transmitted light, then for reflected light where the manipulation is simpler.

7.2 The DIC microscope

In the basic DIC microscope the necessary splitting and recombining of the beam is achieved by devices known as Wollaston prisms, one mounted before the condenser serving as a beam splitter, and a second one after the objective acting as a beam combiner. A Wollaston prism consists of two geometrically similar wedges of doubly-refracting material, quartz or calcite, cut so that their optical axes are at right-angles one to the other. A beam of plane-polarized light entering the prism at 45° to its axis will be split by the prism into two mutually perpendicularly polarized beams, separated by a small angle (see *Figure 7.4*). In a DIC microscope (see *Figure 7.5*) a polarizer is placed in the light path, followed by a Wollaston prism in the first focal plane of the condenser, set at 45° to the plane of polarization. Light passing through each point within the condenser aperture will be split by the prism into two beams; the members of each pair will be made parallel to one another as they leave the lens, and separated by a distance shown, much exaggerated, as *x* in the diagram. These beams will pass through closely adjacent regions of the object. On entering the objective lens the beams will be brought to a focus in the back focal plane, where a second Wollaston prism will redirect each pair into a common path. Since the two members of each pair of beams derive from a common origin in the first focal plane of the condenser (and in Köhler illumination, therefore, from a common point on the lamp filament), they are coherent and thus capable of interference. The pairs of beams, still polarized at right-angles to one another, will then pass through a second polar, the analyser, crossed with respect to the polarizer, and with its plane of polarization again at 45° to the planes of polarization of the two beams. Here the components of the two beams vibrating in the plane of polarization of the analyser will be recombined, and allowed to interfere.

The system as described requires a Wollaston prism to be fitted in the back focal plane of the objective, a location which is not normally accessible for the insertion of accessories. Microscopes built on these principles require a set of special objectives for DIC; the prisms are fixed and the objectives will therefore be unsuitable for general work. Nomarski's contribution to the DIC microscope was a modification of the Wollaston prism to allow it to be placed at a greater distance from the objective lens than the focal plane. This is achieved by cutting one of the parts of the Wollaston prism at an angle oblique to its optical axis. The effect of the modifications is that the prism functions as if it were positioned in the focal plane of the lens, even though it is situated some distance further away (see *Figures 7.6* and *7.7*). In this figure, the path of one of the two beams through the Nomarski prism appears to defy the rules of refraction as they are normally understood. It is, however, correct. This apparently anomalous behaviour is a result of the fact that in anisotropic materials, in which refractive index varies with the direction of the light, the ray direction is not necessarily perpendicular to the wave normal (the normal to the vibration direction of the wavelets). Snell's law applies to wave normals, which are equivalent to ray directions in familiar isotropic materials where refractive index is constant in all directions. When a ray passes through an anisotropic crystal in certain directions, the angular difference between the ray direction and the wave normal can be quite large. This is an

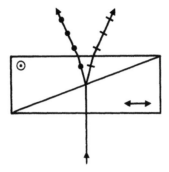

Figure 7.4: Schematic diagram of a Wollaston prism.
This diagram shows the angular separation of the two emergent beams which are polarized in mutually perpendicular directions. The arrow in the lower half of the prism indicates the optic axis.

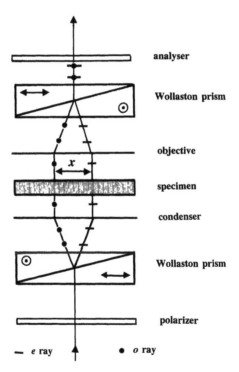

Figure 7.5: An interference microscope.
This is an interference microscope such as that devised by Smith, in which the beams are divided and recombined using Wollaston prisms mounted in the first focal plane of the condenser and the back focal plane of the objective. The separation between the beams (x) as they pass through the specimen is relatively large, with consequent doubling of the image.

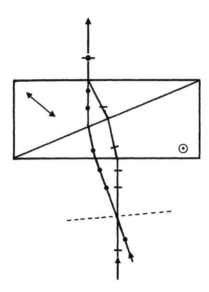

Figure 7.6: Nomarski's modification of the Wollaston prism designed for use with an objective lens.

Inclination of the angle of optic axis in the upper half of the quartz wedge results in the projection of the apparent plane of recombination of the two beams outside the prism itself. This permits the prism to be mounted behind the objective lens while the plane of recombination lies in the back focal plane. Notice that the plane of the wavefront (indicated by the dashed line) is not exactly parallel to the prism surface.

important factor in the design of the Nomarski prism, producing the effect shown in the diagram.

Manufacturers of microscopes differ in the ways in which they have incorporated DIC into their instruments, particularly with respect to the location of the second Wollaston prism. In some instruments these are permanently mounted within a set of special objectives, while others provide the prisms, again one for each objective, mounted in sliders which can be inserted into slots either in adapters fitted between standard objective lenses and the nosepiece, or within the nosepiece itself. An alternative system, again allowing the objectives to be used for other techniques, has one common Wollaston prism mounted in a slider which can be inserted into the microscope tube, and which is designed to serve all objectives. It may be made adjustable up and down, so that the point of intersection of its pairs of beams coincides with the back focal planes of objectives of different focal length. Where the prisms are mounted in sliders, provision is usually made for them to be moved laterally by means of a screw. This alters the relative thicknesses of the upper and lower components of the cemented wedges through which the beams pass, and allows contrast to be adjusted (see below); a similar effect may also be achieved by slight rotation of the polarizer. Members of each pair of beams will encounter differing optical paths due to variations in refractive index and thickness of components of the object. Where both paths through an area of the object are equal, both beams remain in phase and, as would normally occur with crossed polars, the field is maximally dark. Where optical path-length differences are present, due to steps or gradients in refractive index or thickness, one beam will be advanced or retarded in phase with respect to the other. The optical path between members of a pair of beams can also be altered by sliding the second Wollaston prism laterally to the optical axis, in one or other direction in its adjustable mount, thus advancing one or the other beam with respect to its counterpart. The phase difference between two beams presents image features in polarization col-

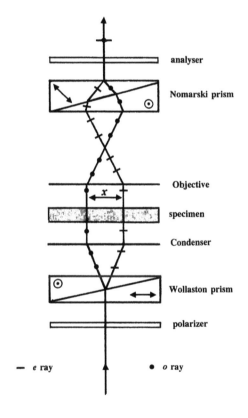

Figure 7.7: The Nomarski differential interference contrast microscope.
Note that the system is symmetrical above and below the specimen. The separation (x) between the pairs of beams as they pass through the specimen is smaller than the distance that the object lens is able to resolve and hence no double image is observed.

ours, as described in Chapter 5. Again as in polarized-light microscopy, small differences in optical path can be accentuated by the insertion of a full-wave plate (first-order red plate), an image in shades of grey thus being transformed into colour. A good series of papers on the DIC microscope and its applications have been published by Lang (1968, 1969, 1971).

7.3 The transmitted-light DIC image

Compared with phase contrast, DIC images have higher resolving power, not least because they do not possess the halo which surrounds all contrasted features in phase contrast. Moreover, the technique has extremely shallow depth of field – a characteristic which in some circumstances might be considered to be a disadvantage, but which does make it possible to isolate features lying in one plane within the object by so-called optical sectioning. A further useful characteristic is that DIC is able to form good images of relatively thick objects, whereas for phase contrast to operate at its best the object must be extremely thin.

However, images from DIC, while appearing 'realistic' at first glance, can be considerably more difficult to interpret than those from phase contrast because of the azimuthally directional nature of the optical system. Consider a simple rotationally-symmetrical object such as a sphere. This will not appear symmetrical in the image: in the direction in which the beams are sheared its edges will appear as fine lines or be virtually invisible, while in the other axis one edge will appear bright and the opposite one dark (see Frontispiece). Unless the observer is already familiar with the structure of the object from other techniques, phase contrast especially, it will not be possible unambiguously to describe the shape of this object. It will be helpful to make use of the microscope's rotating stage, if fitted, in order to study the object independently of the directional nature of the imaging technique. Another serious artefact, which arises from the 'shadowing' effect, is what is often described as the 'three-dimensional' appearance of the image. This frequently misleads observers into believing that the image displays true three-dimensionality in the object, whereas this is far from being true. Based on this misapprehension, several generations of students now believe that living cells have the appearance of a fried egg! (see *Figure 6.8c*). It should be remembered that DIC presents features in the image in relief based on their optical path differences, and that in transmitted light these path differences arise from a combination of actual geometrical path lengths and refractive index differences. The nucleus in the centre of the image of the cell is in fact an area where the cell's contents have higher refractive index, and it does not necessarily project beyond its surrounding cytoplasm.

7.4 DIC in reflected light

In comparison with transmitted-light DIC, the construction and operation of the equipment, and even the interpretation of the images, are simpler for DIC used in reflected light, where the objective lens acts also as the condenser. Apart from the simpler procedure of setting up the necessary Köhler illumination for reflected light, the DIC system requires only one Wollaston prism to serve the functions of beam splitter and beam combiner. When this is placed in (or effectively in) the back focal plane of the objective lens, it will simultaneously be situated in the first focal plane of the illuminating lens (condenser). In order to minimize the effect of reflections from the illuminating light, the prism may be mounted at a small angle to the horizontal; in other respects the system and its setting-up are similar to those for transmitted light.

For opaque objects, the commonest type studied by epi-DIC, the image can be taken as a true three-dimensional representation of the surface with just one proviso: correct setting of the Wollaston prism is necessary in order to make clear the distinction between raised and lowered regions (see Frontispiece).

7.5 Setting-up DIC for transmitted light

A transmitted-light microscope equipped for Köhler illumination is needed, with the following accessories:

- polarizer in a suitable rotating mount, located before the condenser
- strain-free condenser fitted with Wollaston prisms appropriate for objectives
- strain-free objectives
- Wollaston prisms to suit objectives
- analyser fitted in the microscope body following the objectives
- full-wave plate (optional)

1. Remove polarizer, analyser, full-wave plate and both Wollaston prisms from the light path. If the second Wollaston prism is fixed within the objective lenses, select an objective of low magnification which is not fitted for DIC, otherwise select the lowest magnification objective for which a DIC prism is available.
2. Set up the microscope carefully for Köhler illumination in bright field using a stained specimen.
3. Exchange specimen for one to be examined by DIC.

4. Insert polarizer and analyser and ensure that they are crossed (i.e. the view through the microscope should be maximally dark). By convention, the vibration direction of the polarizer should be East–West (i.e. left to right), and that of the analyser North–South.
5. Insert the appropriate Wollaston prism after the objective or, where they are integral, change to an objective equipped with a Wollaston prism.
6. Insert the appropriate prism beneath the condenser.
7. If the objective-lens Wollaston prism has an axial (up-and-down) adjustment, use this to produce a field of view of uniform shade of colour or greyness.
8. Adjust the objective-lens prism sideways by means of the screw on its slider, and observe the range of contrast available. Where this prism is fixed, slightly rotate the polarizer away from its crossed position.
9. Insert the full-wave plate into the slot provided in the microscope (somewhere between polarizer and analyser) and repeat step 8; consider which settings provide the desired information about the object.

7.6 Setting-up DIC for reflected light

A reflected-light microscope equipped for Köhler illumination is required, with the following accessories:

- polarizer in a suitable rotating mount, situated in the illuminating rays before the objective
- strain-free objectives
- Wollaston prisms to suit objectives
- analyser fitted in the microscope body following the objectives
- full-wave plate (optional)

1. Remove polarizer, analyser, full-wave plate and Wollaston prism from the light path. If the Wollaston prism is fixed within the objective lenses, select an objective of low magnification which is not fitted for DIC, otherwise select the lowest magnification objective for which a DIC prism is available.
2. Set up the microscope carefully for Köhler illumination in bright field.
3. Insert polarizer and analyser and ensure that they are crossed (i.e. the view through the microscope should be maximally dark). By convention, the vibration direction of the polarizer should be East–West (i.e. left to right), and that of the analyser North–South.
4. Insert the appropriate Wollaston prism at the objective or, where they are integral, change to an objective equipped with a Wollaston prism.
5. If the Wollaston prism has an axial (up-and-down) adjustment, use this to produce a field of view of uniform shade of colour or greyness.

6. Adjust the Wollaston prism sideways by means of the screw on its slider, and observe the range of contrast available. Where this prism is fixed, slightly rotate the polarizer away from its crossed position.
7. Insert the full-wave plate into the slot provided in the microscope (somewhere between polarizer and analyser) and repeat step 6; consider which settings provide the desired information about the object.

References

Lang W. (1968) Nomarski differential interference microscopy. I Fundamentals and experimental designs. *Zeiss Information* **70**, 114–120.

Lang W. (1969) Nomarski differential interference microscopy. II Formation of the interference image. *Zeiss Information* **71**, 12–16.

Lang W. (1971a) Nomarski differential interference microscopy. III Comparison with phase contrast. *Zeiss Information* **76**, 69.

Lang W. (1971b) Nomarski differential interference microscopy. IV Applications. *Zeiss Information* **77/78**, 22–26. These were republished in one Zeiss reprint (number S41–210.2–5–e).

Pluta M. (1993) *Advanced Light Microscopy,* Vol. 3, *Measuring Techniques.* Elsevier, Amsterdam.

8 Fluorescence Microscopy

In 1904 the German microscopist August Köhler was studying the use of ultraviolet light for increasing the resolution of the microscope. He noticed that some objects emitted visible light when irradiated with invisible short-wave ultra-violet. This emission of light is the phenomenon now called fluorescence. The absorbed radiation interacts with some molecules; a photon, absorbed by an atom of the material, causes an electron to move from the lowest energy level (the ground state) to a higher level (an excited state). This is an unstable situation and after a very short time (in the order of 1×10^{-9} sec) the electron spontaneously returns to the ground state, with the emission of a photon (see *Figure 2.8*). A related phenomenon which has not been adequately exploited in microscopy occurs when the time for the electron to return to the ground state is measured in seconds; this is called phosphorescence.

It is characteristic of fluorescence that the emitted radiation has a wavelength peak which is both lower in intensity than that of the exciting radiation and is at a longer wavelength than that of the excitation. This is often known as the 'Stokes shift'. The plots of wavelength and energy of excitation and emission show, however, that they overlap to some extent, a fact which is of importance in the practical choice of filters for use in fluorescence microscopy. *Figure 8.1* illustrates the Stokes shift for the compound fluorescein isothiocyanate (FITC); the excitation range is between approximately 450–500 nm with a maximum at 496 nm in the blue. The emission, however, has its maxiumum in the yellow/green region at the longer wavelength of 518 nm. For practical use with current fluorochromes the exciting radiation wavelength may lie between 300 and 700 nm, that is, from the near ultraviolet throughout most of the visible range.

Fluorescence is of great value in microscopy, largely because of its sensitivity, since the presence of a very few fluorescing molecules may be detected with ease. As the background, composed of the non-fluorescent material, is dark, fluorescence microscopy is obviously a very effective way of generating contrast and often the fluorescence microscope is used for this purpose alone. The sensitivity of the technique has been increased by the use of fluorescent probes, where the fluorescing component is linked to a specific antibody. Another use of fluorescent probes depends on their

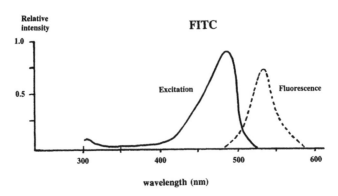

Figure 8.1: The Stokes shift.
The Stokes shift illustrated for the compound fluorescein isothiocyanate (FITC); the excitation range is from c. 450–500 nm, with a maximum at 496 nm in the blue region. The emission, however, has its maxiumum in the yellow/green region at the longer wavelength of 518 nm and has a lower intensity than the exciting radiation.

rapid response, compounds having now been devised which allow cell biologists to detect and measure transient events which have a very short time scale.

8.1 Types of fluorescence

The fluorescence shown by many natural compounds when they are excited with relatively short wavelengths (approximately 365 nm) is called *autofluorescence*. Substances which show autofluorescence may prove troublesome in applications of fluorescence microscopy, since the generalized autofluorescence may mask another desired type of more specific fluorescence. Common examples of autofluorescent materials are fluorite, chlorophyll, amyloid and collagen.

Some of the components found in biological tissues (e.g. adrenalin, noradrenalin and histamine) although not autofluorescent themselves, may become fluorescent after chemical treatment with compounds such as formaldehyde. This is usually known as *induced fluorescence*. One of the earliest applications of fluorescence was to use strongly fluorescent substances (such as the dye acridine orange) to bind to a particular substrate in the tissue, thereby enabling it to be located with the fluorescence microscope. Dyes used in this non-specific way are known as *fluorochromes*. It is analogous to the standard process of staining with coloured dyes, but has the advantage that many colourless, or almost colourless, substances which could not be used as dyes are strongly fluorescent and may be used for fluorochroming. Because of the great sensitivity of fluorescence and the fact that fluorescence microscopy provides a self-luminous image on a dark

Table 8.1: Commonly used fluorochromes

Fluorochrome	Excitation maximum (nm)	Emission maximum (nm)
Acridine orange (bound to DNA)	502	526
Allophycocyanin (APC)	650	661
Aminoactinomycin D	555	655
7-Amino-4-methylcoumarin-3-acetic acid (AMCA)	317	445
BCECF	505	530
Calcium green	505	532
Cascade blue (Pyrenyloxytrisulphonic acid)	376, 399	423
DAPI	350	470
Eosin	525	545
Ethidium bromide	510	595
Formalin-induced fluorescence (FIF)	405	435
Fluorescein isothiocyanate (FITC)	496	518
Hoechst 33258 (bound to DNA)	346	460
INDO-1	350	405–482
Lissamine rhodamine B200	575	595
Lucifer yellow VS	428	533
Nile red	515–530	525–605
Pararosaniline (Feulgen)	570	625
Phycoerythrin R	480, 565	578
Propidium iodide	536	617
Rhodamine 123	511	534
Rhodamin B	540	625
SNARF	563	639
Tetramethyl rhodamine isothiocyanate (TRITC)	554	576
Texas red	596	615

Many complex fluorochromes are usually known only by their abbreviated names or acronyms as above.

·background, fluorochromes may often be detected at very low concentrations and this has led to some applications where they are introduced into living cells as vital stains. *Table 8.1* gives a reference list of some of the fluorochromes in current use, together with their excitation and emission maxima. Details of many current fluorochromes will be found in Brelje *et al.* (1993).

The major drawback of most direct fluorochromes is their lack of true chemical specificity. The technique of *immunofluorescence* has changed this and introduced great specificity; the linking of specific antigen with antibody, after one or the other has been labelled with a fluorescent molecule, allows visualization of their location in tissues. Many variants of this technique have been developed in recent years and it is now used extensively, along with other microscopical methods (e.g. confocal microscopy), to study the location of cellular components, such as actin filaments, and also in nucleic acid hybridization studies.

Fluorescent compounds are now frequently being used in cell biology as markers of physiological changes. This is because, as mentioned above, fluorescent probes (often of great chemical complexity and referred to by acronyms such as FURA-2 or INDO-1) have been developed which are sensitive to such rapid and transient events as changes in the ratio of free to bound calcium ions or changes in the pH of the cytosol. Currently, techniques are being developed to use multiple fluorescent probes on the same cell, coupled with excitation in sequence with several different wavelengths. The collection and storage of the corresponding fluorescent images and their possible recombination allows the location of various cell organelles, and the ratios of some intracellular ions in their various states, to be measured (Shotton, 1995).

Most fluorescing substances are degraded to some extent by the energy of the exciting radiation and their fluorescence will thus fade. It is important, therefore, to minimize unnecessary exposure of the object to the radiation, for example by blanking off the beam except when the image is being observed or recorded. In some cases fading may be so severe that the image can be lost even during a photographic exposure!

8.2 The fluorescence microscope

In the early days of fluorescence microscopy, transmitted light was used with the addition of a glass filter to the illumination path so as to isolate a given range of excitation wavelengths. Such 'excitation filters' were wideband short-pass filters (see Section 8.4) and the exciting radiation was usually provided by a high pressure mercury arc. Although there was little problem in exciting adequate fluorescence from the rather non-specific fluorochromes then in use, there was a problem in removing from the light path the superfluous exciting radiation which tended to swamp the wanted emitted fluorescence. This removal was attempted by including a long-pass 'barrier filter' in the light path above the specimen. In some early objectives which were made specifically for fluorescence microscopy, the yellow barrier filter was cemented on to the front element of the objective itself, where it also prevented image degradation from fluorescence of the lens components themselves. Later fluorescence microscopes placed the barrier filter in a separate mount above the objective, enabling the filter to be changed according to the wavelength of the exciting radiation, and, by removing it, allowing the objective to be used as a conventional objective.

It was soon realised that many of the problems of transmitted-light fluorescence microscopy could be reduced by using dark ground, with the excitation radiation concentrated on the specimen at such a degree of obliquity that none of the exciting radiation falls within the acceptance angle of the objective. However, small amounts of this exciting radiation will be scattered by the specimen and directed into the objective, as in normal dark-ground imaging, and the use of a barrier filter is thus still important. The result of this procedure is a considerably darker background than with the transmitted-light system, allowing the detection of weaker fluorescence and the attainment of higher contrast in the image. However, the use of dark ground had the disadvantage that, as the objectives usually had a high numerical aperture, the condensers had to be cardioid or bicentric reflecting types, which must be used in immersion contact with the underside of the slide and are not easy to focus and centre. Such disadvantages, however, are relatively minor and are outweighed by the increase in efficiency provided by transmitted dark-ground fluorescence as compared to the alternative method of direct illumination. This approach to fluorescence microscopy was much used in diagnostic microscopy.

The real stimulus for fluorescence microscopy was provided in the late 1960s by the work of Ploem, who introduced the extensive use of epi-fluorescence with a standard vertical illuminator fitted with interchangeable dichroic mirrors. A dichroic mirror reflects through the objective, on to the specimen, almost all of the incident light with a wavelength shorter than a pre-determined value. At the same time it allows the shorter wavelength radiation (the emitted fluorescence) to pass through and form the image. When a vertical illuminator fitted with a dichroic mirror is used the objective acts as its own condenser, so there are fewer alignment problems, and all the excitation is directed downwards on to the area to be studied. The exciting radiation falls on to the surface of the specimen so that attenuation by absorption or scattering in the object is minimized and the fluorescence of opaque specimens can be studied just as easily as those which transmit light. There is yet another advantage in the use of epi-illumination, as the transmitted-light path remains available for an independent alternative method of direct illumination to be used at the same time. Good general references for fluorescence microscopy are the books by Ploem and Tanke (1987), and Rost (1991, 1992, 1995). The newer applications are considered in Herman and Lemasters (1993).

8.3 Light sources for fluorescence

It is important for obtaining sufficient contrast by fluorescence that the exciting radiation should be within the correct range of wavelengths for the fluorochrome in use and that the radiation should be of high intensity. This latter requirement may sometimes restrict the choice of light source to strong line emitters, that is, those that have high levels of energy output at certain well defined wavelengths which stand out from a less intense continuum of radiation. In current practice three major types of source are in use, namely tungsten halogen lamps, mercury arcs and high pressure xenon arcs. Lasers are now often used for excitation of fluorescence in confocal microscopy; interested readers will find a good introduction in Brelje (1993).

Tungsten halogen lamps provide a continuous spectrum extending from about 400 nm to above 900 nm, with virtually no peaks (see *Figure 8.2a*). It is obvious that such excitation will not be of use for fluorochromes which require significant excitation in the ultraviolet or near ultraviolet range. Tungsten light sources are, however, suitable for fluorochromes such as FITC (fluoroscein isothiocyanate), which have their excitation maxima at longer wavelengths, and these light sources have the advantage that they are cheap and can be used for other techniques of microscope illumination.

The xenon arc is another light source which has been used as excitation for fluorescence. This light source emits a continuous spectrum from ultraviolet to red but has strong peaks in the far-red and infra-red (see *Figure 8.2b*) regions. For this reason the exciting filter set must contain suitable red-suppressing filters. The xenon arc has the disadvantage that its life is relatively short and the bulbs are expensive. Since such lamps contain the gas at high pressure, even when cold, they must be in suitable lamp housings and the relevant safety precautions taken in their handling.

The most commonly used light source for fluorescence is the high pressure mercury vapour arc which is available in 50, 100 or 200 W versions. There is a strong continuum in the spectrum of a mercury arc which, however, is characterized by strong emission peaks at 366 nm, 436 nm and 546 nm together with several other lesser peaks (see *Figure 8.2c*). These peaks make this a particularly good excitation source for many different fluorochromes when this lamp is combined with suitable filters. As with the xenon arc, mercury lamp housings should be fitted with adequate heat barrier filters.

8.4 Objectives and filters

Although fluorescence can be observed with ordinary achromat or plan-achromat objectives, for maximal contrast it is advisable to use objectives specifically designed for this method of contrast. The chief problem is in maximizing the amount of exciting radiation and emitted fluorescence which is passed by the objective to form the image. For this reason high transmission through the various components is desirable and the individual components of the objective must, of course, not show auto-fluorescence. For this reason fluorite cannot be used for components of objectives designed specifically for fluorescence microscopy. More impor-

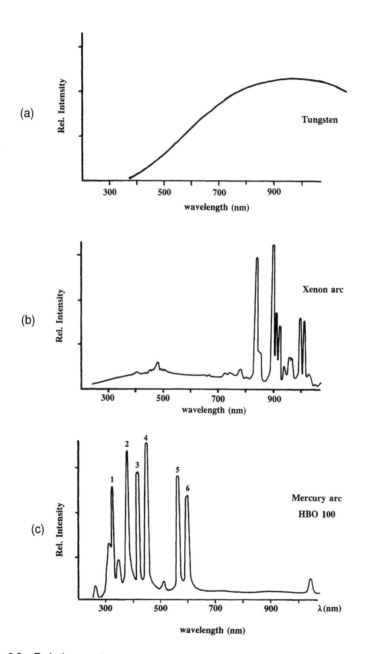

Figure 8.2: Emission spectra.
Emission spectra of (a) a tungsten filament lamp, (b) a xenon arc and (c) a mercury HBO100 arc. Note that the spectrum of the tungsten lamp is continuous, whereas those of the two arcs show distinct peaks. The mercury arc is particularly rich in the short wavelength components.

tantly, however, objectives designed specifically for fluorescence should have a higher than usual numerical aperture for their magnification. This is to achieve maximum image brightness rather than the highest degree of spatial resolution. Since the intensity of light passing through a lens depends on the area of that lens, the intensity is thus proportional to the square of the numerical aperture. In an epifluorescence system both exciting and emitted radiation pass through the objective lens and the intensity of the observed fluorescence will thus be proportional to the *fourth* power of the NA of the objective. Image brightness decreases with increase in magnification: it is in fact inversely proportional to the square of the magnification. For this reason the most intense fluorescence images result from the use of objectives of the highest numerical aperture and relatively low magnification. For this reason objectives in a set intended specifically for use with fluorescence thus have low magnifications and high numerical apertures, often designed to be adjustable for immersion in water, glycerin or oil. For example, a water-immersion objective is available having a magnification of only 40 and a NA of 1.2. The use of immersion helps to maximize the gathered light by reducing the possibility of reflections at the front glass surfaces. Again, in order to maximize image brightness, fluorescence microscopes are often used with low power oculars.

Also important for successful fluorescence contrast is the choice of the excitation and barrier filters and the dichroic mirror which must all be of high optical quality. In modern fluorescence microscopes using epi-illumination, these three components are often combined into a single 'filter block' which forms part of the illuminator. When different fluorochromes which have different excitation and emission maxima are in use, the block may be quickly changed for another fitted with different filters. The use of infinity-corrected objectives allows the simple inclusion of the 'filter block' in the optical path without significant reduction in the image quality. The early excitation filters, sometimes called short-pass or KP (German, kurzpass) made of dyed-in-bulk glass such as the BG12, were 'broad-band' and allowed a relatively large spread of short wavelengths to reach the specimen (see *Figure 8.3a*). Better results were often obtained with glass narrow-band filters. These transmit only a narrow band of wavelengths and are chosen to have their maximum transmission at a single wavelength which is the optimum required for the excitation of a given fluorochrome (see *Figure 8.3b*). Currently the use of coloured glass filters may be replaced or supplemented by an interference filter, which can be manufactured with a much narrower band-pass, in order to make the excitation wavelengths more specific.

Barrier filters (long-pass filters) are placed between the objective and the eyepiece and are designed to block any remaining shortwave exciting radiation but transmit the longer wavelength fluorescence. As with excitation filters, the transmission characteristics of a barrier filter (see *Figure 8.3c*) are chosen with the fluorochrome's specific emission in mind. Each manufacturer provides comprehensive lists of matched excitation

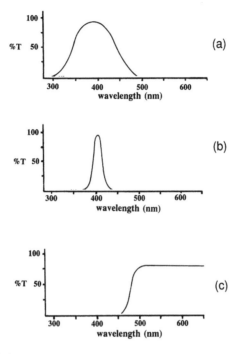

Figure 8.3: Transmission curves.
Transmission curves of (a) a wide-band glass excitation filter such as the BG12 or BG3; (b) a narrow-band filter with maximum transmission at c. 400 nm; (c) a typical 'long-pass' filter used as a 'barrier' filter.

filters, dichroic mirrors and barrier filters to suit different types of autofluorescence and specific fluorochroming; as new fluorochromes are constantly being developed, it is desirable to consult the relevant manufacturer's current literature for the specification of suitable filters for any particular use. In addition, the barrier filter is an essential component in any fluorescence microscope system in order to protect the observer's eye from damage, should any unwanted short wave radiation manage to pass through the microscope.

Dichroic mirrors (more correctly called dichromatic beam splitters) are composed of a complex system of multiple layers of metals, metal salts and dielectrics which have been vacuum-deposited on to thin glass. These coatings are designed with thicknesses and refractive indices to enhance or block transmission and reflectance at specific wavelengths. They are much more efficient than, for instance, a simple semi-transparent reflector surface. With this latter, at least 50% of the exciting radiation will be lost by passing straight through the glass reflector and similarly, another 50% of the emitted fluorescent radiation will be lost before forming the image. This dual loss means that the maximum efficiency will only be approximately 25%. A specially coated dichromatic beam splitter, on the other hand, is capable of passing approximately 90% of the incident exciting radiation down into the objective and transmitting a similar amount of the emitted fluorescence, resulting in very much brighter images.

Fluorescent images, even using epi-illumination with these highly efficient dichromatic mirrors, are often lacking in brightness, which may prove a problem in recording them. It is usually possible to obtain excellent 35 mm photomicrographs on colour film balanced for daylight. The 35 mm format is preferable to the use of larger film, since with the latter the intensity at the film would be considerably lower due to the inverse square law, often requiring unacceptably long exposures. It is now usual to add a TV camera or a photomultiplier to the microscope system to display, and possibly to process and store the image by means of a computer system. It is possible to increase the brightness and contrast by the use of electronic image intensification which is built into the camera itself, but it is now more common to use computer-assisted low light imaging with fluorochromes. A comparison of the suitability of standard video, silicon intensified target (SIT) and CCD cameras for this purpose will be found in the paper by Shotton (1995). Provision of permanent hard-copy output is now easy with the use of the new dye-sublimation colour printers linked to the computer; these allow very high quality colour prints to be obtained quickly and at reasonable cost.

References

Brelje TC, Wessendorf MW, Sorenson RL. (1993) Multicolor laser scanning confocal immunofluorescence microscopy: practical application and limitations. In *Methods in Cell Biology* (ed. B. Matsumoto) Vol. 38. Academic Press, San Diego, pp. 98–193.

Ploem JS, Tanke HJ. (1987) *Introduction to Fluorescence Microscopy* (RMS Handbook no. 10). Oxford University Press, Oxford.

Rost FWD. (1991) *Quantitative Fluorescence Microscopy.* Cambridge University Press, Cambridge.

Rost FWD. (1992) *Fluorescence Microscopy,* Vol. 1. Cambridge University Press, Cambridge.

Rost FWD. (1995) *Fluorescence Microscopy,* Vol. 2. Cambridge University Press, Cambridge.

Herman B, Lemasters JJ. (1993) *Optical Microscopy. Emerging Methods and Applications.* Academic Press, San Diego.

Shotton DM. (1995) Electronic light microscopy: present capabilities and future prospects. *Histochem. Cell Biol.* **104**, 97–137.

Technical brochures by manufacturers such as Leica, Nikon, Olympus and Zeiss are often excellent sources for technical details on this aspect of contrast enhancement.

9 Enhancement of Contrast in the Image

It is obviously desirable to achieve the necessary contrast in the microscope itself, by enhancing either an amplitude or a phase image by using suitable optical means. There are instances, however, where all the contrast which may be introduced by altering the conditions of microscopy is still not sufficient. It may then become necessary to add further contrast to the image after it has been produced by the microscope. For many years the only possible recording technique was drawing, either free hand or by means of an optical aid such as a camera lucida. Here, the selective enhancement of contrast is easy, using the standard techniques of an artist, such as colour, emphasis with shading and the use of darker pencils or Indian ink (Bracegirdle and Bradbury, 1995).

When a drawing is used to record the image there are several other advantages not related to contrast enhancement. It is possible to synthesize, in one drawing, information from several planes of focus within one specimen, information from several specimens of the same object, and also to emphasize features considered to be of special importance.

9.1 Photographic techniques of contrast enhancement

The invention of photography in the middle of the nineteenth century led to the use of photomicrography for recording microscope images. Photomicrographs have the advantage that they may be viewed by several persons at the same time and they are permanent and convenient, often saving many pages of verbal description. They do suffer from the disadvantage that each micrograph represents one particular appearance, chosen by an individual microscopist, which therefore necessarily represents that individual's conception of the organization of the specimen and may indeed not be representative of its true character. The advantages of photomicrography in the present context are that photographic techniques may be used to adjust image contrast very considerably. It is desirable, however, to ensure that as much of the contrast needed in the image is achieved by the optical arrangements of the microscope, before resorting to photographic manipulations.

The contrast of an image recorded on to a photographic negative is largely governed by the characteristics of the film itself and the development used to process the film. When a negative has been produced there is still further scope to alter contrast during the printing stage which produces the positive from the negative. If colour positive or negative film is used, the possibilities of contrast manipulations at the photographic stage are much reduced.

9.2 Film choice, negative development and printing

When light affects a photographic emulsion a number of the silver halide crystals are affected and can be transformed into silver metal by the developer, the nature of which can affect markedly the contrast of the resulting negative. The characteristics of the film/developer combination may be assessed by exposing successive areas of the film evenly to light at a constant intensity and aperture, but with exposures which are successively doubled. After development under controlled conditions the optical density of each negative is measured and plotted graphically against the logarithm of the exposure. This was first done by Hurter and Driffield and the resulting curve (see *Figure 9.1*) was formerly called the 'H & D' curve, but is now termed the 'characteristic curve'. This curve has a flattened 'toe', a straight line portion and a 'shoulder' representing the greater exposures. Even when there has been no exposure to light there is some density, causing the toe of the curve not to start at zero, but at some point above this, a point which represents the density of the film base itself plus that of the silver grains formed by action of the developer even on unexposed silver halide grains. This density (base + fog) results in the toe of the curve having a small portion running parallel to the zero point on the y-axis. The slope of the straight line part of the curve is a measure of the contrast of the negative. This was formerly called 'gamma', but contrast is now expressed as 'contrast index' (CI). This is defined as the slope of a straight line drawn from a point 0.2 density units above the base fog level to a point 2.0 units above this level. Details of the full photographic significance of contrast index will be found in text books on photography, for example that by Langford (1986). For the present purpose it is sufficient to understand that the contrast index of a given film may be modified considerably by development.

Films themselves are formulated by the makers for specific purposes; one intended for general use (film A in *Figure 9.1a*) would have a much lower contrast index (as shown by the lesser slope of the relevant part of

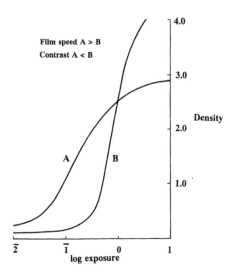

Figure 9.1:   Characteristic curves of two films.
The characteristic curves of two films with differing speeds and contrast indices. Film A is intended for general use whilst film B, of much higher contrast, is intended for scientific use in recording objects of low contrast.

the characteristic curve) than film B in *Figure 9.1*, which could have been specifically formulated with a much higher contrast index for scientific work.

It is possible to use a film of intrinsically high contrast and vary the development so that the contrast index achieved is suitable for the need of the moment. In epi-illumination, the contrast produced by the microscope is often high; transmitted-light dark-ground images are also high in contrast. For these it is often unnecessary to boost the contrast, indeed, quite the reverse. With these techniques it will usually be found that a contrast index of between 0.5–0.7 is sufficient. This range of contrast indices is easily achievable with a film such as Kodak T-Max 100 developed to various degrees in Kodak HC110 developer. The contrast of an image may require boosting photographically by developing to about CI 1.0 for a stained histological specimen when studied with a contrast filter; normally stained specimens usually require a CI of 1.5. To achieve this contrast, and that of 2.0 or even 2.5 (which might be needed if the specimen is a polished metal or a ceramic which has an intrinsically low contrast), a different film should be used. A typical choice might be Kodak Technical Pan, whose CI may be varied between 0.5 and 2.5 by choice of a suitable developer concentration and development time, together with alteration of the film speed rating. Details of suggested starting points for experimentation along these lines will be found in the book by Bracegirdle and Bradbury (1995).

If the object is coloured then, as discussed on page 29, contrast may be enhanced on the negative by the use of a suitable colour filter; such gains may be further increased at the printing stage by use of a paper of high contrast, if necessary. It is far better, however, to try to gain sufficient contrast on the negative to give a satisfactory print on paper of normal contrast. This type of paper gives the greatest latitude for the production of a full range of tones and thus conveys the maximal amount of information. Details of such photographic methods of contrast enhancement will be found in Bracegirdle and Bradbury (1995) and in standard texts on photomicrography such as those by Loveland (1970) and the Kodak booklet (Delly, 1988).

9.3 Image enhancement by video techniques

Photography is now supplemented by video recording of microscopical events as they happen, incidentally adding the dimension of time to the scientists' records and opening up other possibilities of contrast modification. Parpart (1951) and Flory (1951) recognized the value of television for increasing contrast in a microscope image, but their approach was overlooked for some time. Possibly this was due to the ease and success of photomicrography; in addition, the video images of that time were restricted in size by the available monitors and by the loss of fine detail due to the coarse scans. Also, there were no adequate video recorders available at that time. Today cameras and recorders are reasonably cheap, easily available and of high quality. Consequently, video microscopy is now commonly used for recording purposes as an alternative to photomicrography. Good surveys of simple equipment for this purpose are provided by Dodge *et al.* (1988) and Strange (1992). Television is now widely used as a method of contrast enhancement especially for studies of transient events in living cells. Most recently of all, microscopical images have been captured by a video camera and subsequently digitized for storage in computer memories. With such an image it is possible to perform mathematical operations on the original image (represented in the computer by a large matrix of numbers) and thus alter the contrast, reduce random 'noise' in the image and sharpen the boundaries between objects and their background. Such image processing is now fast becoming routine in both conventional and confocal microscopy (Bradbury, 1988).

Early video cameras used a tube to convert the image into an electronic signal; more recent cameras replace this with a solid-state device or 'chip' using semi-conductor technology. It is now common for the video camera to use a single chip or charge-coupled device (CCD) instead of a vacuum tube with its target and scanning beam. These CCD cameras are lighter, smaller and require less power than the conventional tube cameras; they have low geometrical distortion.

As the electronics of video cameras allow control over the contrast and the black level, it is thus possible to use video technology to enhance the contrast of microscopical images. At the same time, any rapid changes in the image due to transient events in the specimen may be recorded for later playback and analysis, possibly in slow motion. Inoué (1981) used video to improve the images in polarized light microscopy and in differential interference microscopy.

Allen and his co-workers (Allen *et al.*, 1981a,b) also applied video to images from the polarized light microscope and to differential interference contrast microscopy; these methods became known as AVEC-POL and AVEC-DIC, respectively. The essential feature of video-enhancement is that operation of the 'gain' (amplification) control of the camera increases both the contrast *and* the brightness of the resulting video image. The 'black-level' control of the camera can then be used to reduce the brightness on the monitor to a normal level, while leaving the image with increased contrast. This technique clearly increases contrast derived, not only from features in the specimen, but also from other sources (e.g. uneven illumination). These defects can be removed by subtracting an image of a field of view which does not contain a specimen.

9.4 Image modification by digital techniques

The use of digital techniques in handling the microscope image has increased steadily over the last 15 years or so. This may be attributed largely to the increase in the availability of small, very powerful digital computers which possess large amounts of memory. At the same time there has been a proliferation of easy-to-use computer software using proven mathematical techniques to alter and manipulate the image. As a necessary preliminary to modifying images by computer manipulation, the image must first be digitized and stored in the computer memory.

The signal from a typical television camera is an analogue signal; this means that as the beam scans across one line of the image the voltage representing the signal will vary continuously. It is possible to 'sample' the signal electronically at regular intervals and convert the signal voltage at those times into a number. Thus, instead of a continuously varying signal as the line scans across the image, we have a series of numbers, each representing the voltage at that particular time in the line scan. These numbers may then be stored in the memory of a digital computer and, by a reverse process, subsequently used to recreate the image. The image becomes broken up into a series of discrete picture elements or 'pixels'.

Whether the image is taken from a tube-type TV camera or from a CCD device, the signal from each pixel (which is proportional in strength to the brightness of the image at that point) is represented by a number. The size and number of the pixels in an image will, of course, determine its spatial resolution, but we must also consider the number of grey levels which the device is capable of reproducing. Our eyes are not capable of appreciating more than about 30 different shades of grey, but for contrast enhancement and image-processing purposes we may wish to work with such subtle differences that 256 grey levels are required in the digitized image. Such an image would therefore need 8 bits (1 byte) to encode a single pixel. If we have an image of 256 × 256 pixels (now considered a relatively coarse spatial resolution) we will need 262 144 bytes to store the image. If we are prepared to digitize in such a way that only four different grey levels are represented then only 2 bits would be needed for each pixel and the memory storage requirements for a whole image can be reduced by a factor of four. If we wish to show the image in terms of black or white alone, (i.e. a binary image) then only 1 bit is needed to store the

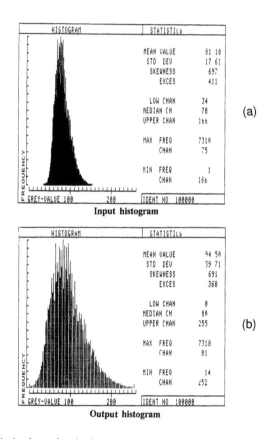

Figure 9.2: Analysis of grey level values.

(a) The printout from an image analyser of a frequency plot of the grey level values for the pixels of a low-contrast image; note that they occupy only a narrow range of 'bins' of grey values. (b) Is a similar printout from a high-contrast image, where the values for the pixels cover a wide range of grey values.

information as to whether the pixel is black or white. Now that large amounts of computer memory are available and relatively cheap, such considerations of image compression are less important than they were only a few years ago. This subject is rapidly expanding and the interested reader is referred to the book by Russ (1990) and an excellent review by Shotton (1995).

9.5 Contrast enhancement by manipulation of the grey-level histogram

Once we have a digital value for the intensity (usually with an 8-bit digitizing system from 0 for black to 256 for white) of each pixel in the image the values may be sorted by the computer into 'bins' of an intensity histogram. The range of values and the number of pixels in each bin give a large amount of information about the image. If the pixels are all in a narrow range of bins, then the image has a low contrast (see *Figure 9.2a*); conversely if the pixels occupy a large, widely scattered number of bins then the image will have a high contrast (see *Figure 9.2b*). There may also be two clearly separated peaks, one corresponding to the darker pixels representing an object, the remainder the lighter background. Such a clear-cut distinction will then allow the operator to instruct the computer to consider only those pixels in a certain range and make measurements on those. This is the operation of 'segmentation' or 'thresholding' essential in

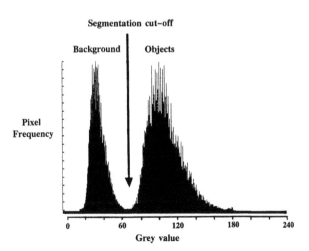

Figure 9.3: Segmentation of grey values.
   The operation of 'segmentation' by which an image can be separated into regions of different degrees of grey values in order to allow independent analysis of the features. There are two peaks of grey values lying on either side of a segmentation cut-off threshold.

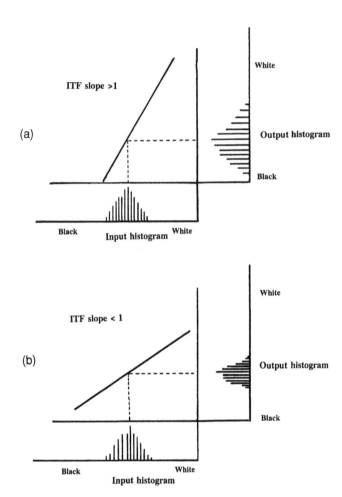

Figure 9.4: The effect of using transformation algorithms on grey level histograms to manipulate contrast in an image.
In (a) the intensity transfer function (ITF) has a slope of greater than 1, hence the grey levels in the output histogram are expanded to cover a wider range than those in the input histogram, and contrast is increased. In (b) where the ITF slope is less than 1 the reverse is true.

all image analysis procedures (see *Figure 9.3*).

More importantly, however, it is possible to transform the shape of the histogram and write a 'new' image histogram by applying what is called an 'intensity transfer function', or ITF, to the histogram. Such an ITF may or may not be linear. By the use of such ITFs it is possible to compress or expand a histogram representing the pixels of an image. It is also possible to reverse the contrast completely, in effect changing a positive image into a negative one. *Figure 9.4a* shows the transformation effects of using a linear ITF with a slope of greater than 1. In this case, where there is an expansion of the output histogram (as compared with the original input), there is an increase in contrast; conversely, when the ITF has a slope of less than 1 (see *Figure 9.4b*), the contrast of the output image will be decreased. In practice, this operation may be achieved by the use of pre-designed 'look-up' tables (or LUTs) which speed up the computation process (Adler, 1996; Shotton, 1993).

The human eye is capable of assessing and recognizing, as separate, about 20–30 different shades of grey. It is, however, much better at the perception of colour, and for this reason the changes of contrast introduced by LUTs in the computer are often represented by so-called 'false colours' where a colour is assigned by the computer to a given range of grey values. Such techniques are frequently used in the presentation of astronomical images and those produced by tomographic scanning.

References

Adler J. (1996) The use and abuse of look up tables. *Microsc. Anal.* **51**, 5–7.

Allen RD, Strömgren-Allen N, Travis JL. (1981) Video-enhanced contrast differential interference microscopy: a new method capable of analyzing micro-tubule related motility in the reticulopod network of *Allogromia laticollaris. Cell Motil.* **1**, 291–302.

Allen RD, Travis JL, Strömgren-Allen N, Yilmaz H. (1981) Video-enhanced contrast polarization (AVEC-POL) microscopy. *Cell Motil.* **1**, 275–289.

Bracegirdle B, Bradbury S. (1995) *Modern PhotoMICROgraphy* (RMS Handbook no. 33). BIOS Scientific Publications, Oxford.

Bradbury S. (1988) Processing and analysis of the microscope image. *Microscopy* **36**, 23–39.

Delly JG. (1988) *Photography Through the Microscope* (9th edn). Kodak, Rochester.

Dodge AV, Dodge SV, Jones K. (1988) An introduction to video recording at the microscope. *Microscopy* **36/1**, 43–53.

Flory LE (1951) The television microscope. *Cold Spring Harbor Symposium* **16**, 505–509.

Inoué S. (1986) *Video Microscopy.* Plenum Press, New York.

Langford MJ. (1986) *Basic Photography* (5th edn). Focal Press, Oxford.

Loveland RP. (1970) *Photomicrography*, Vols I and II. John Wiley & Sons, New York.

Parpart AK. (1951) Televised microscopy in biological research. *Science* **113**, 483–484.

Russ JC. (1990) *Computer-assisted Microscopy: the Measurement and Analysis of Images.* Plenum Press, New York.

Shotton D. (1993) An introduction to digital image processing and image display in electronic light microscopy. In *Electronic Light Microscopy* (ed. D Shotton). Wiley-Liss, New York, pp. 39–70.

Shotton D. (1995) Electronic light microscopy: present capabilities and future prospects. *Histochem. Cell Biol.* **104**, 97–113.

Strange A. (1992) Silicon and silver - video enhanced microscopy - photographing the video image. *Microscopy* **36/8**, 643–649.

Appendix
A Vector Theory Approach to Phase Contrast

The following approach largely follows that of Barer (1959). Mathematically, a vector is a quantity which has a magnitude and a direction. Thus, the phase and amplitude of a beam of light may conveniently be represented in this manner as a line (see *Figure A1a*), whose length OA is proportional to the amplitude and whose direction represents the phase of the vibration (which is the reference for all other beams to be considered). The intensity of the beam is given by $(OA)^2$. Any phase change to a beam will be represented by a vector forming an angle ϕ with OA. If this incident beam passes through an absolutely transparent object then the vector of the transmitted beam may be represented by a line Op, where p lies on the circumference of a circle with radius OA (see *Figure A1b*). If the transmitting object is partially absorbing then the transmitted vector Ov will be shorter, as in *Figure A1c*. It thus follows that all perfectly transparent objects will be related to vectors whose ends fall on the circle with radius OA, and mixed refracting and partially absorbing objects will have vectors which terminate in this so-called 'object circle'.

Readers will remember that vectors may be added by the parallelogram rule which states that "the sum of two vectors is the diagonal through O of the parallelogram of which the two vectors, when represented by lines through O, form adjacent sides". In the case of our perfectly transparent object above, the transmitted beam (Op) can be represented by the sum of OA and a second vector Ap created by the object (see *Figure A2*). This second beam Ap is, of course, the light diffracted by the object which fills the back focal plane of the objective. The incident beam OA and the diffracted beam from each element in the object pass on to recombine with the incident beam and so form the image. If the system were perfect the light distribution in the image would be represented by a vector circle the 'image circle', in this case identical with the object circle. *Figure A3* shows two points in a transparent object which differ only in refractive index or thickness and which are imaged by a perfect system. The incident beam is OA and the two resultants are Op and Op^1, with phase changes ϕ and ϕ^1 respectively, both on the circumference of the object circle which in this case coincides and is identical with the image circle. This means that the objects are invisible and there is no contrast. In practice, of course, the optical system is not perfect, as a result of aberrations in the lens and due to restricted numerical aperture, so that there may then be a shift of ob-

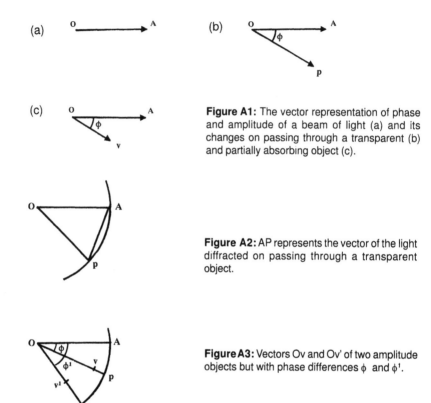

(a)

(b)

(c)

Figure A1: The vector representation of phase and amplitude of a beam of light (a) and its changes on passing through a transparent (b) and partially absorbing object (c).

Figure A2: AP represents the vector of the light diffracted on passing through a transparent object.

Figure A3: Vectors Ov and Ov' of two amplitude objects but with phase differences φ and φ'.

ject and image circles with the introduction of contrast but with loss of resolution of detail in the image. With amplitude objects, such as two particles, the transmitted beams differ according to the absorption of light by the particles and may be represented by the the vectors Ov and Ov^1 (see *Figure A3*); these differ in length, with the result that their intensities $(Ov)^2$ and $(Ov^1)^2$ also differ. These differences are, however, independent of the phase differences φ and $φ^1$.

In phase contrast, differences of phase are introduced between the direct and diffracted beams passing through the system. A phase change of λ/4 is equivalent to one of 90° which may be represented in vector notation simply by rotating the vector through this angle. Thus, after passing through the object the direct light may be represented by the vector OM instead of OA (see *Figure A4*); the image is now formed by OM and, as before, the diffracted light Op. The resultant of OM and Ap may be found by the parallelogram rule by drawing MP parallel and equal to Ap and joining OP. Thus $(OP)^2$ is equal to the intensity of the image of that particular object element, represented by p. In the ordinary transmitted light microscope, the original image point intensity was $(Op)^2$ which was equal

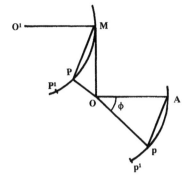

Figure A4: The vector (OM) of direct light which has had its phase changed by 90 degrees. The image is formed by OM and the diffracted light Op, the result of which is (OP). (OP)² is obviously less than either (OA)² or (OM)² and hence there is now amplitude contrast.

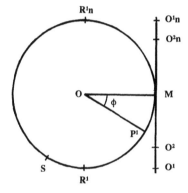

Figure A5: A simplified construction for the vector explanation of phase contrast.

to the background intensity $(OA)^2$ and there was no amplitude contrast. In the phase-contrast microscope with a phase change of $\lambda/4$, the intensity of the image point is now given by $(OP)^2$ which is obviously less than either $(OA)^2$ or $(OM)^2$. The object point appears darker than the background, and refractive index variations and thickness variations which govern the degree of phase change are thus converted into variations in intensity, and contrast has been achieved. Similarly, for another point p^1 on the object circle the intensity of the new image point will be given by $(OP^1)^2$ and so the new image circle has its centre at O^1 and has a radius of O^1M.

In conventional microscopy the object circle coincides with the image circle with a common centre at O; in phase-contrast microscopy the image circle centre is shifted, although the origin from which the intensities are measured remains the same. Since the image and object circles are identical apart from this displacement of their centres, the geometrical construction may be simplified (see *Figure A5*). A single circle may be taken to serve for both object and image, simply shifting the origin of the vector from O to a new origin O^1. In positive phase contrast, where the direct light is advanced in phase by $90°$, the origin of the vector is now at O^1 as a result of rotating OM about M by $90°$, so moving the origin *below* the line OM. For negative phase contrast the vector origin would be shifted *above* the line OM to a new origin at O^1n. From *Figure A5,* it is clear that when the phase of the direct light is advanced to shift the origin from O to O^1, the intensity of all points such as p^1 on the quadrant of the circle MR^1 will be less than the background intensity $(OM)^2$; thus, for values of the phase change ϕ up to 90° a phase-retarding detail should appear darker than the background, producing positive phase contrast. It is worth noting that if ϕ exceeds 90° (e.g. when the object point lies at S on the circle in *Figure A5*), then the contrast would be reversed since the intensity given by $(O^1S)^2$ is now greater than that of the background $(O^1M)^2$. If the direct light is retarded by 90°, then the new origin of the vector is O^1n and we have negative phase contrast and points represented by p^1 will appear brighter than the background. Those details which are represented by points on the quadrant of the circle R^1nM will now appear darker than the background.

It should be noted that the intensity of the direct light may also be altered. If a fraction $1/N$ of the direct light is transmitted then the origin of our vectors shifts to O^2 or O^2n of *Figure A5*, where $O^2M = 1/\sqrt{N}$. This will reduce the overall intensity, but at the same time enhance small differences of relative intensity or contrast. A full treatment of the effect on contrast of phase plates with different absorptions is given in the reference by Barer.

Reference

Barer R. (1959) Phase, interference and polarizing microscopy. In *Analytical Cytology* (ed. RC Mellors) (2nd edn). McGraw Hill, New York, pp. 169–272.

Index

Modern PhotoMICROgraphy

B. Bracegirdle & S. Bradbury
respectively Cheltenham, UK; and University of Oxford, UK

A completely new practical guide to photomicrography and a valuable companion volume to *Scientific PhotoMACROgraphy* by Brian Bracegirdle.

"This has been a pleasure to read and review and can be recommended to both the true amateur and professional alike who wish to further their knowledge of, this art and practice in a truly delightful but authoritative and factual way." J.A. Dutton "A concise but readable handbook covering all aspects of modern photomicrographic practice....thoroughly recommended." Spike Walker, Microscopy and Analysis, January 1996

Contents

Obtaining the image; Imaging methods in current use; Recording the image using graphics methods; Recording the image in monochrome; Recording the image in colour; Special problems and techniques; Publishing the results; Manufacturers and Suppliers.

Of interest to:

All who wish to record photographic images, whether novices or experienced workers.

1859960901; 1995; Paperback; 112 pages

Microscopy of Textile Fibres

P.H. Greaves & B.P. Saville
respectively MICROTEX; and Huddersfield University, UK

An up-to-date practical guide to the properties and characteristics of textile fibres, with clear advice on sampling, specimen preparation and examination procedures.

"This is a well researched, well documented, well presented book.." Aslib Book Guide

Contents

Introduction; Fibre identification; Fibre measurement; Polarised light microscopy; Special preparation techniques for light microscopy; Other light microscopical techniques applied to fibres; Scanning electron microscopy; Transmission electron microscopy; The identification and quantitative analysis of animal fibre blends.

Of interest to:

Textile technologists; Fibre scientists; Microscopists; Forensic scientists; Materials analysts.

1872748244; 1995; Paperback; 112 pages

Scientific PhotoMACROgraphy

B. Bracegirdle
Cheltenham, UK

A detailed practical guide to choosing the correct equipment and methods for both transmitted-light and reflected-light photography.

"...will benefit all microscopists ...Its format is clearly outlined, easy to follow, and quickly directs the reader to successful macrophotographic applications, removing the trial and error approach." *Scanning* "So comprehensive and up-to-date that anyone buying it will be assured of a plethora of excellent advice." *The Photographic Journal*

Contents

The scope of the process; Obtaining the magnification; Working with transmitted light; Working with reflected light; General remarks on illumination and exposure; Estimating exposure in macro-range photography; Recording the image.

Of interest to:

2nd year undergraduates and above; any researcher using the microscope at low resolution.

187274849X; 1994; Paperback; 120 pages

ORDERING DETAILS

Main address for orders

BIOS Scientific Publishers Ltd
9 Newtec Place, Magdalen Road,
Oxford OX4 1RE, UK
Tel: +44 1865 726286
Fax: +44 1865 246823

Australia and New Zealand
DA Information Services
648 Whitehorse Road, Mitcham, Victoria 3132, Australia
Tel: (03) 9210 7777
Fax: (03) 9210 7788

India
Viva Books Private Ltd
4325/3 Ansari Road, Daryaganj, New Delhi 110 002, India
Tel: 11 3283121
Fax: 11 3267224

Singapore and South East Asia
(Brunei, Hong Kong, Indonesia, Korea, Malaysia, the Philippines,
Singapore, Taiwan, and Thailand)
Toppan Company (S) PTE Ltd
38 Liu Fang Road, Jurong, Singapore 2262
Tel: (265) 6666
Fax: (261) 7875

USA and Canada
BIOS Scientific Publishers
PO Box 605, Herndon, VA 20172-0605, USA
Tel: (703) 661 1500
Fax: (703) 661 1501

Payment can be made by cheque or credit card (Visa/Mastercard, quoting number and expiry date). Alternatively, a *pro forma* invoice can be sent.

Prepaid orders must include £2.50/US$5.00 to cover postage and packing
(two or more books sent post free)